NOT NOW TOMORROW

ima nai ashita

A true story by an Australian civilian nurse, from the Government Hospital in Rabaul, who was held prisoner with her colleagues in New Britain and Japan following the Japanese onslaught of Rabaul in 1942

Alice M Bowman

DAISY PRESS

First Published 1996 by DAISY PRESS
PO Box 144
BANGALOW NSW 2479
AUSTRALIA

Researched, edited and produced by Claire Deglon Marriott
© Drawings Graham Marriott 1996

Typeset in CG Times
Printed in Australia by DLT Printing Sydney

National Library of Australia
Cataloguing-in-Publication data

Bowman, Alice M (Alice Mary), 1912-
Not Now Tomorrow = ima nai ashita

Bibliography
ISBN 0 646 20360 6

1. World War, 1939-1945 - Prisoners and prisons, Japanese.
2. World War, 1939-1945 - Personal narratives, Australian.
3. Prisoners of War - Australia - Biography. 4. Nurses - Australia - Biography. 5. Women prisoners - Japan - Biography. 6. Women prisoners - New Guinea - Biography.
7. Rabaul (Papua New Guinea) - History - Bombardment, 1942.
I. Title II. Title: ima nai ashita.

940. 547252092

TABLE OF CONTENTS

THE AUTHOR

Alice Mary Bowman (Bowie) was born in 1912, in Longreach, Queensland. She grew up in the far west under the harsh conditions of Queensland's Channel Country. Her early education was conducted by correspondence, supervised by a Governess, and in her later years she attended boarding school. After training for secretarial duties, Bowie chose to pursue a career in nursing and gained her General Nursing certificate from Maryborough Hospital and her Midwifery certificate from Cairns Hospital. Early in 1939 she was accepted on the staff of the European Hospital in Rabaul, New Guinea.

When Rabaul was invaded and occupied by Japan in the Second World War Bowie and her colleagues became prisoners of war and were held in captivity for three and a half years.

After her recovery from this ordeal, Bowie ran Sister Bowman's Day Nursery in Brisbane. In 1951, while working with the Brisbane District Nurses' Association, Bowie married Gordon Déglon, who was a returned AIF veteran of the Second World War. Bowie worked at Tenterfield and Wagga Hospitals before she and her husband travelled around the world, finally settling in South Africa. South Africa was the birthplace of Bowie's husband.

Bowie continued her nursing into her seventies. After the death of her husband in 1977, although always a loyal Australian, Bowie carried on living at her home in Hillcrest, Natal, surrounded by many friends from her nursing years. She is devoted equally to her companionable dogs and her lavish garden, which abounds with innumerable varieties of Bougainvillea reminiscent of her native Queensland.

Personal liberty is the paramount essential
to human dignity and human happiness.

Bulwer-Lytton

PRISONERS OF WAR from RABAUL

CIVILIAN
ADMINISTRATION NURSES from NAMANULA HOSPITAL

Joyce Oldroyd-Harris	(Oldroyd)
Joyce McGahan	(Joyce/Mac)
Grace Kruger	(Grace)
Alice Bowman	(Bowie)
Jean McLellan	(Liklik)
Dorothy Maye	(Maisie)
Mary Goss	(Mary)

CIVILIAN
METHODIST MISSION NURSES

Dorothy Beale	Dora Wilson
Jean Christopher	Mavis Green

AUSTRALIAN ARMY NURSES

Kathleen Parker	(Kay)	Lorna Whyte	(Whytie)
Eileen Callaghan	(Cal)	Daisy Keast	(Tootie)
Marjory Anderson		Mavis Cullen	

OTHER CIVILIANS

Mrs Kathleen Bignell (Plantation owner - New Britain)
Mrs Etta Jones (American Schoolteacher - Aleutian Islands)

ACKNOWLEDGMENT

I sincerely thank Gordon's daughter Claire in the singular responsibility she undertook to prepare my manuscript for publication; without her enthusiasm, dedication and ghost-writing Not Now Tomorrow would never have gone to print.

My gratitude goes to Graham, Claire's husband, for his staunch support and for his effort in capturing the period with his drawings. To my dear friends Joyce and Bill, whose assistance has been invaluable to Claire, goes a special word of acknowledgment, also to Len Slack for his contribution and use of his father's photographs; and many, many thanks to Ben, Claire's son, and to Peter of Direct Litho Techniques for positive and generous support with printing and preparation of photographs, drawings and maps. A final word of thanks to the Sacred Heart Mission in Sydney for making available archival photographs, and to Margaret Thompson of the Australian War Memorial, Canberra, for her initial encouragement in the project.

Recognition to the old barnacle.

Bowie Déglon

Not Now Tomorrow is written under my maiden name.

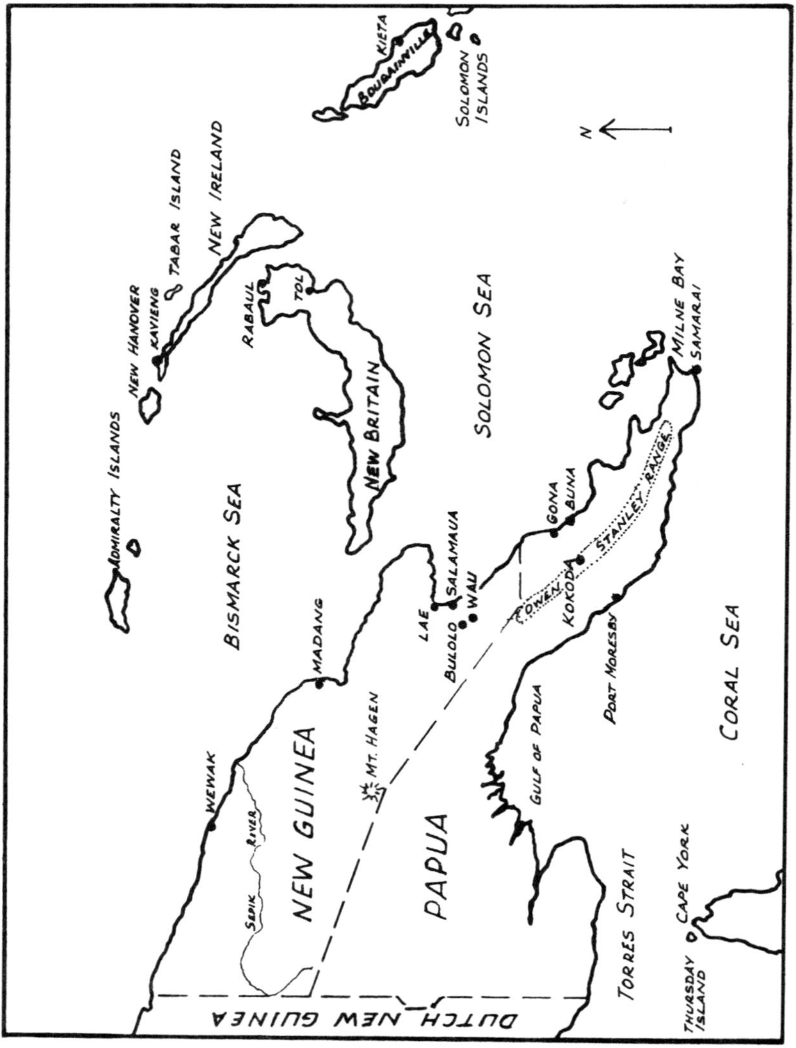
ADMIRALTY ISLANDS
NEW HANOVER
KAVIENG
TABAR ISLAND
NEW IRELAND
KIETA
BOUGAINVILLE
SOLOMON ISLANDS
N
BISMARCK SEA
RABAUL
TOL
NEW BRITAIN
SOLOMON SEA
WEWAK
MADANG
LAE
SALAMAUA
WAU
BULOLO
GONA
BUNA
KOKODA
OWEN STANLEY RANGE
MILNE BAY
SAMARAI
NEW GUINEA
SEPIK RIVER
MT. HAGEN
PAPUA
GULF OF PAPUA
PORT MORESBY
CORAL SEA
TORRES STRAIT
CAPE YORK
THURSDAY ISLAND
DUTCH NEW GUINEA

PROLOGUE

When I began my nursing training Australia was grappling with the adversity of the Great Depression. This disastrous economic collapse was world wide and affected the whole framework of society. Unbelievable numbers were out of work and the subsequent struggle to buy even the bare necessities of everyday living created untold hardship; few escaped the serious worries of those days.

In America, where it all began, confidence was gradually being restored by strong government action following the election of President Roosevelt. In Germany, the crippling effects of the depression began to ignite embers of political dissent, which were stealthily being fanned by that infamous opportunist and leader of the Nationalist Socialist Party, Adolf Hitler, a man who preached peace while preparing for war. And in Australia in the thirties foreboding talk of the growing unrest in Germany could be heard. Another world war?

When old soldiers gathered uneasiness was often expressed about Australia's isolation from Britain and our proximity to the Far East, although, in reality little was known about our neighbours to the north, the Japanese in particular. Could there possibly be a threat to Australia's unending and unprotected coastline? The Japanese were on the side of the Allies in the First World War and it was not a consideration that Australian soil might be endangered from that quarter, accordingly, Japan did not figure noticeably in Australian conversation.

Australia's association with the peoples of the mystical East was limited to the small communities of Chinese living in this "wide brown land". The Chinese came to Australia in great numbers during the last century to seek their fortune on the goldfields and many of their descendants can be found today running small businesses. In days long gone city dwellers enjoyed purchasing fresh vegetables from neighbourhood Chinese gardens.

In happier times too, it was not uncommon for prosperous Australians to take an ocean voyage to the Orient mainly visiting the fascinating ports of Singapore, Hong Kong and Shanghai. Rarely was Japan sought, though, with hindsight, tourists would not have learned much about that country's inscrutable people from such brief visits.

Without a great deal of thought, the Japanese were viewed as being somewhat primitive and regarded only as a nation which exported cheap goods in the line of textiles, crockery and toys. Some people who considered themselves better informed categorically stated: "The Japs are good at imitating imported, manufactured goods and making cheap reproductions on a small scale and, of course, they have the fishing industry, but nothing much else is going on in those small islands". Surely the greatest understatement and misinterpretation of all time!

Looking back, it seems strange that there could have been so much ignorance and complacency surrounding the Japanese. As it later transpired it was not only in Australia that Japan was seriously underestimated, but in America and Great Britain and most of the vast Asia-Pacific region.

Looking back even further to the beginning of Japan's recorded history, it is intriguing to uncover a truculent country with centuries of civil unrest. Intense rivalry between powerful rural families in the pursuit of supremacy led to constant feuding and brought about a dominant warrior class society among the Provincial clans. From this origin came the evolution of Japanese military power.

Under their Shogun leaders, the strength and influence of the Provincial clans escalated, causing the decline of the Imperial Court of the Emperor and the creation of a *Shogunate* government. The Shoguns were forceful military dictators, who exercised authority mercilessly through their Samurai administrators, however, power struggles persisted. In the seventeenth century the ruling Shogun introduced a radical policy of national seclusion in the hope of eliminating unrest caused by foreign intrusion and, along with it, Christianity, which was considered a threat to the unity of the people. For two and a half centuries under this edict Japan was closed to foreign ways and stability was maintained.

Social and political events, in the nineteenth century, led to the abdication of the Shogunate regime and brought about the restoration of the divine Emperor as supreme head of government. Under a new Constitution the warrior class nobility were financially compensated for loss of status and their loyal Samurai (trained only to be warriors) were absorbed into the civil service, the police force and a new national army. A period of enlightenment followed and, with the adoption of a synthetic Western civilisation, feudal ways were irresolutely cast aside and dramatic changes spread across Japan.

In its long and curious history Japan had never suffered defeat from an invasion of its shores; the Japanese believed they were protected by the Gods and held devout faith in a contrived 'myth' of invincibility. Not surprisingly, the government's emerging military leaders covertly devised a stratagem which, they believed, would consolidate Japan as a perpetrator, never to become a victim.

Rumours circulated during the thirties of Japanese interest in South East Asia and the Pacific; among Australians there was no grave alarm. Surreptitiously, with the almost unopposed occupation of Manchuria in 1931, territorial expansion of Japan began; relentless aggression in Eastern China followed. A veil of secrecy shrouded the mysterious Land of the Rising Sun and obscured the paramount objective of that remote island nation. Could we, then, not be excused for failing to grasp the true significance of the steadily increasing power in government of the Japanese militarist extremists?

Meanwhile people everywhere laboured on. About two years after I had completed my training I decided that a change of scene, preferably a change overseas, would be a good idea and would broaden my experience. Discussions with friends revealed that they too had itchy feet and needless to say we all shared the same problem, no money! Opportunities for Australian nurses seeking appointments in the British colonies were highly favourable and many of the girls expressed a preference for either Singapore or India. Applications for these places had to be sent to England, which I thought somewhat involved, so I applied for a position nearer home; I could always move further afield later.

My choice was the Australian Mandated Territory of New Guinea. Tropical islands had a beckoning aura of adventure and romance about them, in those days especially, when little had changed in the way of life since contact with the Western world.

Several months passed before an official envelope arrived stamped External Territories, Canberra. I opened this before an interested group of my colleagues and announced, rather smugly, that I had been accepted on the staff of the European Hospital in Rabaul on the island of New Britain. This was early in 1939.

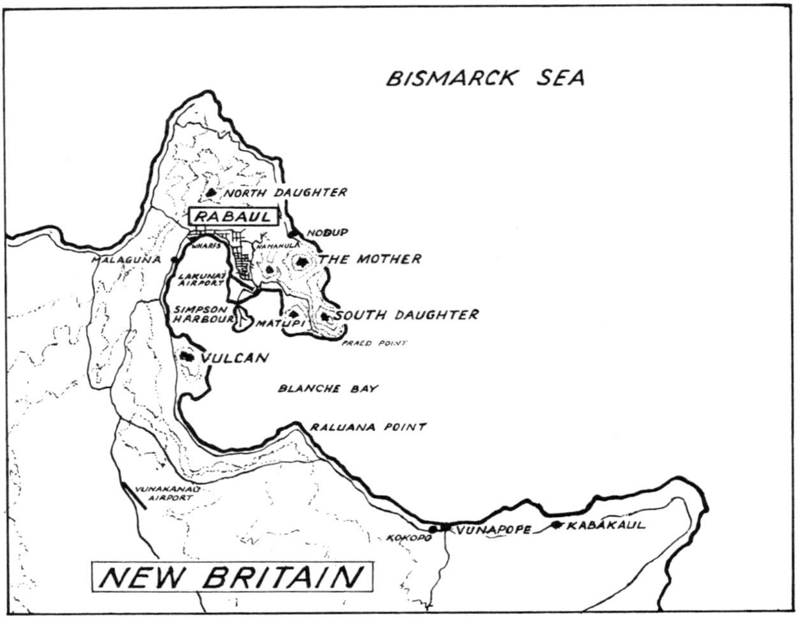

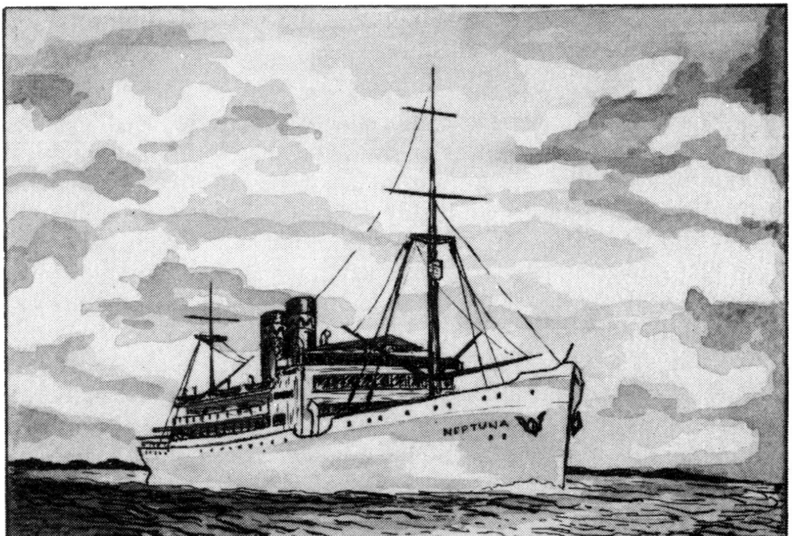

The MV *Neptuna*

1

RABAUL

Bidding farewell to Australia, I set forth on the MV *Neptuna* to take up my new appointment in Rabaul. The *Neptuna* was a handsome ship, one of a number in the Burns Philp fleet running regularly from the east coast of Australia to New Guinea and other exotic places in the Pacific. There were a few new-comers like myself on board, but the majority of passengers were old-timers of the Territory returning home after a visit down south. They had many tales to tell about *their* islands, most of them rather tall, though none the less interesting and very entertaining.

This was a happy voyage. It took about ten days, during which time the attentive crew with some help from the passengers organised lots of activities. In between relaxing, vigorous deck games were played by the energetic; the not so energetic became absorbed in a good book or lounged about in comfortable deck chairs engaging in amiable conversation. Sumptuous meals were served with old world charm in the ship's lavish stained-wood dining room. The atmosphere on board was characteristic of a friendly community with everyone enjoying the company of everyone else; an all round sense of well-being gave to the new-chums a tangible feeling of already belonging to the Territory.

The night we entered the Whitsunday Passage in the Great Barrier Reef was one of those never-to-be-forgotten experiences. The beauty of this area is well known to Australians if only by repute and the claim of a tropical paradise, with jewel-like islands set in glassy turquoise seas, was not an exaggeration. Nothing could be more awe-inspiring under a full moon than to move slowly through the shimmering waters of this narrow, winding passage to the Pacific

Ocean. On this, my first voyage, the Whitsundays remain the highlight, beautiful though the many other islands were.

Our first landfall was Port Moresby, dwarfed by mountainous terrain. The township was cradled in the headland and humid, lifeless air hung low over the sweltering harbour like an all enveloping wet blanket reducing the passengers to limp forms sprawled in canvas chairs along the deck.

'There's not much cargo coming aboard, so we'll soon be pulling up anchor,' announced one of the old hands on returning from a stroll around the ship. Immediately there were audible sighs of relief and signs of animation among the deck chairs and bars; cold beer dominated the conversation.

After rounding the tip of the New Guinea mainland the *Neptuna* called briefly at the tiny, coral strewn, island port of Samarai. Steering a northerly course we cruised through the dotted islands around Milne Bay to the open sea *en route* to Rabaul.

Rabaul, the then centre of administration of the Australian Mandated Territory of New Guinea, rests peacefully on Simpson Harbour at the sheltered end of magnificent Blanche Bay, surrounded by volcanic mountains. The extinct volcanoes of the South Daughter and North Daughter are embraced by The Mother, who dominates the scene. Matupi, rising at the foot of The Mother and Vulcan on the other side of the bay are small, but decidedly active volcanoes and keep steadfast vigil over the entrance to Simpson Harbour. Yet another volcano, though dormant, Rabalanakaia, nestles unobtrusively on the side of The Mother.[1]

On entering Blanche Bay the passengers were on deck, marvelling at the spectacle, when one of the old-timers quite casually remarked to me that residents of this area are no strangers to volcanic activity. Rabaul is, quite literally, built on the edge of the crater of an ancient volcano, he explained, and earthquakes, rumblings and eruptions are a frequent occurrence. The whole bay is a giant caldera, three kilometres wide, and was formed thousands of years ago when the south eastern edge was breached and flooded by the sea.

As we drew nearer, the houses were scarcely visible scattered sparsely among the thick green foliage of the foothills. Almost the whole population of Rabaul must have been on the wharf waving and calling to passengers as the ship came alongside. Ashore, the Customs presented a scene more like a 'welcome committee' than the austere, brusque reception one might have expected. Returning residents were greeted with enthusiasm while officials listened to accounts of the latest news from down south. The officers concerned barely glanced at my luggage and were wishing me a happy stay in the islands when a young man came forward and introduced himself as a member of the Public Health team. John, as he asked me to call him, had been sent to deliver me to the hospital.

Leaving behind the pungent smell of copra, stored in huge sheds beside the wharf, we travelled along a wide tree-lined avenue bordered with hibiscus and croton shrubs. Many of the streets were named after the trees that lined them, John explained as we turned out of Mango Avenue and wound our way up Namanula Hill. The car came to a halt in front of a sprawling old building.

'Here we are, this is Namanula Hospital.'

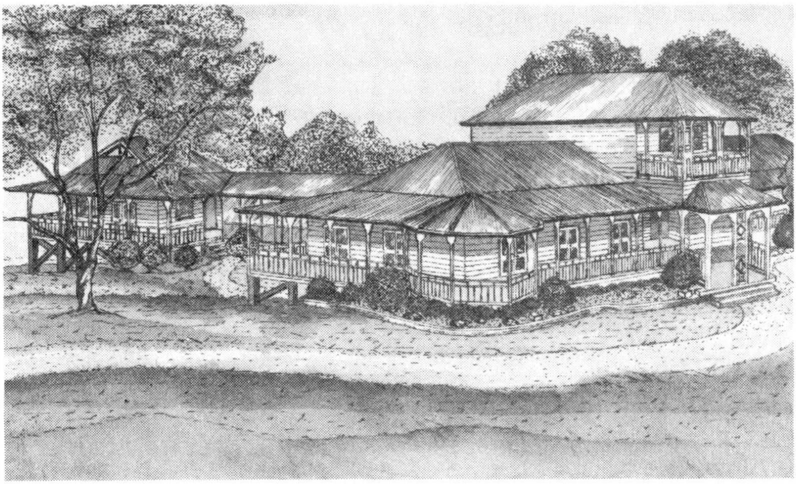

Namanula Hospital

As we went up the steps of the portico entrance to a wide verandah a slight woman in uniform appeared and John introduced me to Miss Thorburn, the Matron of Namanula. Three other Sisters very soon came to meet me, Grace Kruger, Jean McLellan and Joyce McGahan; together we formed the trained nursing staff of the hospital. We were all from Queensland, as was my predecessor who had already left to take up a post in Singapore.

Namanula Hospital had been built by the Germans, who originally settled New Britain, and it passed into Australian hands early in the First World War. The several timber buildings, comprising the hospital, were spread around the site and raised above the ground in the manner of the older houses in Queensland. The wards were spacious with high ceilings and wide doors which opened onto equally lofty, wide verandahs. Huge trees overhung the wide verandahs and filtered the sunlight; these generous old trees and gracious old buildings presented a picture of absolute tranquillity.

The nurses' home, which I found out later was referred to as the House Sister or more correctly *haus sister* was built along the same lines as the hospital and connected to it by glassed-in passage ways. The bedrooms here were spacious as well and filled with heavy dark furniture. However, what really caught my eye and kindled my imagination was the amazing size of the beds which surely must have been brought out from Europe in the last century. They were huge brass four-posters - the likes of which I had never seen - with a raised partition down the middle dividing the enormous mattresses. Later Thorbie, as the matron was affectionately called by the staff, told me that the Germans had used them as hospital beds, although she could not say whether more than one patient shared these monsters. It was not feasible to move such large beds around the ward so more suitable equipment was installed when the Australians took control of Namanula. The controversial beds were relegated to the *haus sister* and I must say when one got used to them they were quite comfortable and definitely roomy.

Impressive too in our quarters were the bathrooms, the *haus waswas*, which were actually large shower rooms because there was no bath. A container for water worked on a system of pulleys and was filled by a houseboy from below; as there was no shortage of labour at Namanula a *waswas* was never a problem.

Soon after settling in I found that it was of prime importance to understand and speak the language of Pidgin. Throughout New Guinea there were hundreds of native dialects, but Pidgin was understood by most groups, and new-comers, including myself, soon mastered it after learning a few native words. It was first in use during German times and a sprinkling of German words remain; its Melanesian words stem from the Kuanua language of the Tolai people in the Rabaul area of New Britain. Many attempts were made by Australian authorities to discourage the use of this Pidgin *English*, as it was considered, among other things, demeaning. However, the vigorous and effective use of the language ensured its survival and it became the *lingua franca* throughout New Guinea. The hospital was called the *haus sik*, and the kitchen the *haus kuk*, and any place where food was served was *place long kaikai*. The favourite food of the natives was the humble *kaukau* or sweet potato, which grows abundantly in the tropics and which was to play a vital role in our own lives at a later date. On hearing the name given to the house where the unmarried - mostly women - Government employees lived, we doubted that this name originated with the natives. Their quarters were known as the *haus virgin*!

Rabaul was a captivating old colonial township and had undergone many changes since it was first settled by the Germans. European settlement on New Britain was founded by a German trading company in 1884 at Kokopo, on the southern coast of Blanche Bay, but because of Kokopo's exposed anchorage a decision to relocate was made in later years to the more favoured site of Rabaul. With its secure, deep harbour, Rabaul - this *place of the mangroves* - was to offer an excellent trading port for the big German companies, which had, by then, become well established. However, trading was enjoyed in the new port for only a very short time before fortunes changed with the defeat of Germany in the First World War.

Quite early in the 1914-1918 war German New Britain surrendered to a small Australian force and that North Eastern part of New Guinea, which was called Kaiser Wilhelmsland by the Germans, fell under the guardianship of the Australian Military. In 1921 the area became the Mandated Trust Territory of Australia, granted by the League of Nations, and Rabaul flourished as the centre of the new Civil Administration.

Many of the Military officers remained and joined the Civil Administration; the first Administrator was the past military leader, Brigadier-General Wisdom. Settlers from Australia flowed in to take up the expropriated German plantations. Others ventured inland, on the mainland of New Guinea, to explore and open up the unknown and hostile interior with its mountainous terrain and almost impenetrable jungle. When the outlying settlements of Salamaua, Wau, Lae, Madang and Kavieng were eventually established hospitals were staffed with doctors, nurses and medical assistants to help in the fight against the terrible diseases of this area, lying just a few degrees below the equator. Malaria, blackwater fever and tropical ulcers, to name only a few, were rife in this humid climate. The battle was ongoing and responsibility for the hospitals at the outstations, as the settlements came to be known, was in the hands of the Matron of Namanula Hospital, as well.

Rabaul did indeed become a busy seaport and the wharves were constantly alive with shipping. The arrival of the big, well-known ships was a social event for the whole town. Fresh food, brought from Australia, was distributed throughout the islands from the Cold Storage, commonly known as the *Freezer* in Rabaul.

Government and privately owned schooners plied between Rabaul and the coastal settlements of New Britain, the New Guinea mainland and the scattered islands of the Bismarck Archipelago, which retained its German name in spite of many name-changes after the Mandate of 1921. Most large plantations in the region operated vessels for trading and collecting supplies, and one could see many a plantation name engraved across the transom of these seaworthy craft.

On the mainland of New Guinea, large transport planes carried goods and materials to the coastal settlements and to the recently discovered goldfields deep in the highlands of the interior. In 1927, Guinea Gold No Liability company posed an ably contested challenge to the bold frontier pilots of its newly formed company, Guinea Airways Limited, when airstrips were adventurously constructed at the goldfields and the seaport of Lae - transporting the heavy mining equipment by air was the only means of getting it to the goldfields. It is claimed that more air freight was lifted from these airstrips than anywhere else in the world in the thirties, particularly when the Bulolo Gold Dredging Company was formed to mine the rich deposits of gold in the Bulolo Valley. Lae was a town literally owned by Guinea Airways and had earned its place on the map as a centre of aviation. It was from Lae that the famous American aviator, Amelia Earhart, and her navigator Fred Noonan took off in 1937 to cross the Pacific on one of the final legs of her round the world flight. Their disappearance without trace has left many controversial theories unanswered to this day. In spite of an immediate, extensive search for sixteen days, by the American Navy and American Airforce, not a single sign of aircraft wreckage could be found.

The airmen of this era were pioneers of aviation, whose skill and expertise did so much towards opening up this rugged country; with the outbreak of the Second World War they were to gain recognition far beyond the boundaries of the Territory, as were the Government District and Patrol Officers. There were no roads into the tough interior or over the high mountains and Patrol Officers performed their duties at great personal risk pushing their way on foot through jungle tracks, gaining expert knowledge of the terrain. The areas patrolled were inhabited by fierce New Guineans, and on many occasions in remote villages Patrol Officers encountered cannibals and head-hunters. In the early days during the search for gold not all fearless adventurers were fortunate to escape the hostility of the highland tribes; some paid the ultimate price.

There was an extensive settlement of Chinese in Rabaul, which I was surprised to find and, in comparison with the size of the other occupied areas, Chinatown was large. The Chinese came to New Britain as indentured labourers brought over by the Germans. Free settlers from China followed and prospered, in spite of many restrictions imposed on them. The shops in Chinatown were fascinating and as Rabaul was a free port many interesting and cheap wares could be purchased. My carved teak chest cost me so little and was a valued possession; within the confines of its camphorwood lining many precious items were saved from spoiling in the dank tropical climate.

Having worked in Cairns in the far north of Queensland, I was accustomed to the hot sultry tropics with frequent bathing and changing of uniform a necessity, and it took only a short time to adjust to the routine of duties at Namanula Hospital. One noticeable difference at Namanula was the abundance of native staff to do many of the tasks junior nurses would have done in Australia. My colleagues at the hospital welcomed me without question, as most people do in the islands, and before long Joyce McGahan and I became close friends. I was introduced to the New Guinea Club, which was the favourite haunt of the residents and where Joyce and I spent many happy hours relaxing under cool Hunter fans swirling from high ceilings. The sporting activities of the Club and popular monthly dances were just some of the social amenities available in this small town with its limited European population.

In those days movies were eagerly awaited by everyone, everywhere, and towns all over the English world had a Regent Theatre for showing them, Rabaul was no exception. It was here, in 1940, that I remember seeing a very young Spencer Tracy in one of my all-time favourite movies, 'Captains Courageous'. The Regent, which was a stately building, was the only picture theatre in town and was converted for use quite often to stage 'live theatre', produced by the Rabaul Dramatic and Musical Society. The Society's Limehouse Theatre was too small to accommodate a large audience and a full house at the Regent was a fitting tribute to the professional performance of the Dramatic Society's many plays, devotedly rehearsed for such long hours.

Life in Rabaul was relaxed and comfortable, having that undisturbed quality of the islands without the pressure of time, and I felt well satisfied that I had made the choice to come to New Guinea. An air of contentment prevailed within the composed atmosphere of the hospital. There were no problems here like those associated with the vast distances of the Queensland outback, where I grew up, and where our nearest Doctor was two hundred and fifty miles away. The

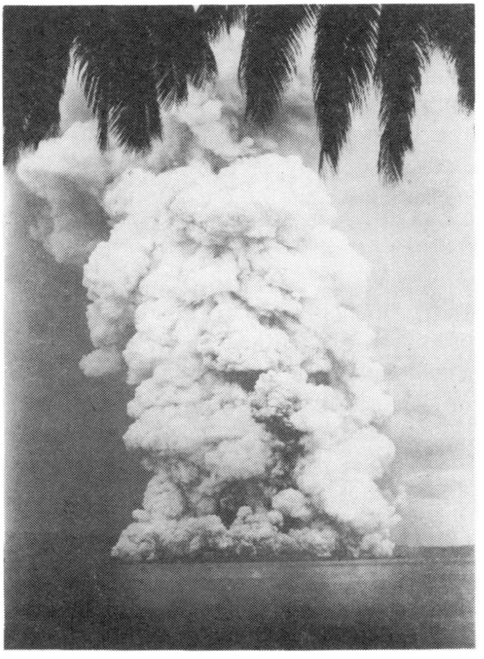

Eruption of Vulcan Island

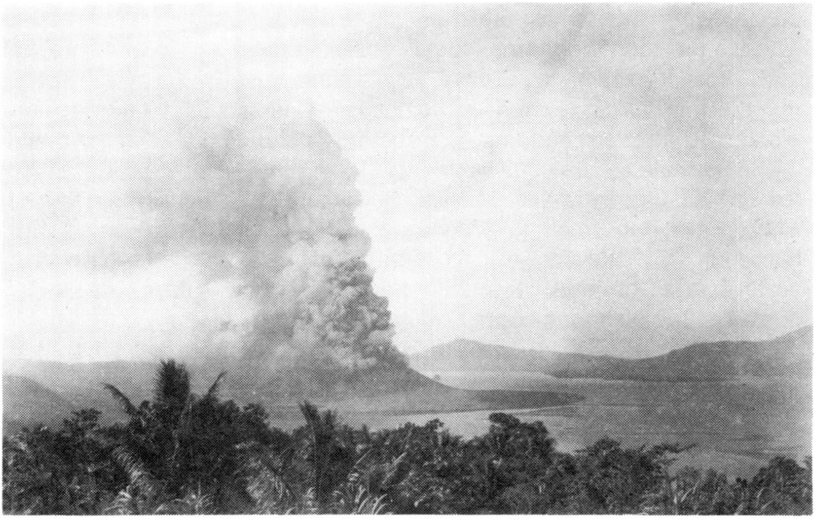

Birth of a volcano - Mount Vulcan

native orderlies were capable and their natural pleasantness made them easy to work with; our only difficulty was in the recruiting and training of native wardresses, female assistants to serve in the Women's Ward.

Namanula Hospital was small by Australian standards. Our male patients were mostly veterans of the First World War who had remained in Rabaul with the Civil Administration and had witnessed close to three decades of seasons in the islands they loved. They were always eager to tell us stories about New Guinea, but the story most favoured, which happened in recent years, was of an event unprecedented in the history of the region. It came to be known as Black Saturday and Sunday and stood as a constant reminder not to be complacent about these lethargic, smouldering volcanoes that create the picturesque and seemingly peaceful scene around Rabaul.

On Saturday, 29th May 1937, flat Vulcan Island began to rise alarmingly out of the sea. Heaving convulsively and groaning ominous warnings the island exploded in violent eruption. Astonished onlookers witnessed the birth of a volcano! Voluminous clouds of glowing pumice and enormous rocks were ejected with such force as to be thrust ten kilometres high. This great eruption threw up a causeway which connected the island to the mainland and devastated all the land to which it joined itself. Natives from nearby coastal villages, who had gathered for a *tabuan* ceremony (a pre-Christian activity not approved of by the missionaries), were trapped and sought refuge in the Mission church. Tragically, more than four hundred Tolais perished when the church collapsed under ten metres of molten pumice. And the land, that settled into a small volcano, forever became a monument over their tomb, and from this time forward was known as Mount Vulcan. The island, Vulcan, was aptly named by the Germans after the Roman God of Fire.

Vulcan continued to erupt sending forth billowing columns of fine ash, which blotted out the sun and turned day into night. Sunday did not see the dawn and further havoc struck when thundering Matupi allied with Vulcan in eruption. Violent storms engulfed the area and the darkness was lit only by streaks of forked lightning; chaos was everywhere. Terrified residents fled to Nodup on the north coast and when this haven became threatened the refugees were hurriedly evacuated from the beach on the ships *Golden Bear* and *Montoro* and as many small craft as could be mustered. Over five thousand Natives, Europeans and Chinese were taken on a hazardous journey to the safety of Vunapope Sacred Heart Mission at Kokopo on the south coast.

When the heaving mountains quietened sufficiently working squads were organised to 'clean up' the town. The destruction caused by the fine volcanic ash, assisted by torrential rain, was unbelievable and two weeks went by before the townspeople and villagers were allowed to return to their homes, only to view with dismay the desolation within and vanquished gardens without. The weight of the ash caused the leaves to fall from the trees and these leafless trees looked on like silent sentinels; palms were so neatly decapitated as though a workman had been busy with his saw.

Two months later, the editorial in the *Rabaul Times* mentioned: "Large areas of pumice still floating in the harbour, streets still lined with huge heaps of volcanic mud and street lights still absent; furtive glances at Matupi and Vulcan sent nerves a-tingle".

There is a geographical fault running across Blanche Bay which causes submarine, volcanic activity. The Tolais had given Vulcan Island the name Rakaia, from their own language, when, in another dramatic chapter in 1878, this doubtful island was thrust up from the sea in a single night. *Kaia* is the native word for supernatural spirits and volcanoes are possessed with very powerful *kaia*!

As time went by nature, ever bountiful in the tropics, came to terms with the harsh surroundings and green shoots appeared through the blackened ground. Nearly a year later, when leaves were growing on the apparently lifeless trees and the first Frangipani bloom appeared, the residents held a celebration dinner dance at the Club. This celebration became an annual event to mark the anniversary of the rebirth of Rabaul, but was abruptly halted in 1942 by the unparalleled occurrence of the Pacific War.[2]

With the gradual build up of events in Europe, which insidiously began with Adolf Hitler's violation of the Peace Treaties (subsequent to the Armistice of 1918) and which climaxed with the German onslaught of Poland, it came as no surprise when World War II was declared on the 3rd of September 1939. I had been in the Territory barely six months. Britain had no choice but to oppose Hitler's aggressive policies if she were to preserve the rights and liberties held dear and not allow the terror of a police state to reign in Europe. Australians everywhere rallied and joined the forces to strengthen Britain's stand.

In New Guinea our loyalty needed no test, the AIF quota set by the Australian Government was filled in record time. A grand, civic parade to honour the men of the New Guinea AIF quota, who were committed to see action abroad, was held before their departure. Our Police Band proudly led the march and the stirring strains of

Land of Hope and Glory, among other sacred airs, resounded through the streets of Rabaul. Many other local citizens, classified by man-power as having essential skills, swelled the ranks of the New Guinea Volunteer Rifles. This voluntary contingent was formed immediately war was declared and was an integral part of the Australian Military Forces. Under the strict terms of the League of Nations Mandate, no military force was allowed in a protectorate territory and Australia had adhered rigorously to this policy; not so Japan, who developed the former German colonies granted to her under Mandate after the First World War. Among these entrusted island groups north of the Equator, the Carolines, Marshalls and Marianas, Japan established military and naval bases for so called 'strategic defence'. The world was to find out later that they were also developed for aggression.

When the second New Guinea AIF quota departed from New Britain's shores, seventy alien internees were transported to Australia with them. Meantime, our lives and our work went on with little difference, the alarming magnitude of the war on the other side of the world was a very long way from us, *longwe tumas* as the natives simply put it.

When Joyce McGahan first came to New Guinea she was on a relief posting at the hospital in Salamaua. The Administration transferred her to a permanent position in Rabaul shortly before my arrival. It was through Joyce that I met Noel Mulvey, who had been in New Guinea for a long time. Noel was a Survey Engineer with the Public Works Department and Joyce knew him in Salamaua when he was surveying a proposed new road from that incredibly small peninsula settlement to Wau, which was twenty miles away up a steep and slippery track and took at least four days to traverse - even by the very fit. Wau was the centre of the Morobe gold mines and inaccessible except by air, as was the gold mine town of Bulolo. Noel and I found we shared common interests and it was not long before we became inseparable companions.

During 1940 Matupi again started rumbling and belching out wisps of grey smoke which persisted continually throughout 1941. Fine grey dust settled everywhere, there was no real escape from it in Rabaul. It reminded me all too well of my childhood in the Channel Country of far western Queensland. The hot dry winds would blow in from the Simpson Desert and sweep along with them the pale orange dust of the parched land; so fine a dust, that it somehow found its way into our home and stifled the air within. The lonely sandstone edifice, with its earth floor, was built on ground level and we were constantly clearing away dust that settled on the window sills and piled up against

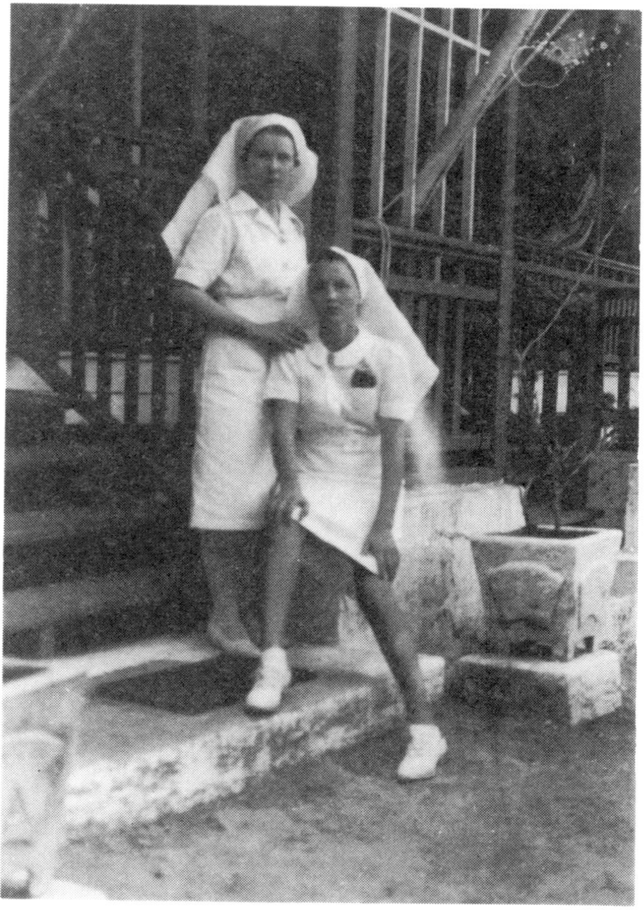

Joyce and myself (seated) at Namanula

the doorways along the verandah. There was nowhere to escape from it in Queensland, either. My parents owned and ran the hotel at Canterbury, one hundred miles west of Windorah and historically known by the locals as 'The JC'. John Costello was a noted pioneer of a legendary era of settlement along Cooper's Creek and the Diamentina, and his initials, carved into a landmark tree, became impregnated forever in the name of the township.

A watchful check on the continual eruptions of Matupi and earthquake activity was now being kept by a seismographic team and their reports were presented weekly in the *Rabaul Times*. The problem was becoming so troublesome that a proposal to move the seat of Administration to Lae on the mainland was confirmed and put into action. The recurring fall-out was a very disagreeable and smelly irritant and the cause of a good deal of corrosion, from the sulphur content, yet we learned to live with it. Soon, we were to have more to be apprehensive of than earthquakes and volcanoes.

It had long been my desire to have my own car to travel about in, and when one of the District Officers was going on leave to Australia I was able to purchase his old Chevy Tourer from him. My driving ability was limited and a few mishaps were encountered during tuition. Memorable among them was the time I drove into the foundations of the nurses' quarters, while parking; fortunately, the foundations were sturdily built and the only damage done was to my car, and my reputation! Eventually it became a great pleasure to drive about the countryside on days off duty.

On many occasions the fall-out from Matupi was evaded when Joyce and I visited the plantation of friends, Keith and Heather Munro, who lived near Kokopo on the south coast. Heather was a trained nurse and did relieving work for us at the hospital; Keith was secretary of the Kokopo Sports Club and, apart from organising regular sporting venues, he introduced Gala days at the Club to raise money for the Red Cross. The Gala days were always well attended, with picnic lunches and sporting activities all part of the enjoyment. There were clowns to entertain the children and lots of interesting stalls, chocolate wheels and raffles. The array of prizes were donated by business people and at one such function Joyce won a bottle of perfume from Davies Drug Store in Rabaul. These charity days were usually rounded off with a dance at the clubhouse in the evening and a good time was enjoyed by everyone.

Community organisations were raising money for the war effort and women all over New Britain were giving their services. Doctor Brennan, our Director of Public Health, was also chairman of the Red Cross Society and under its guidance small groups were formed to train the local people in general nursing and other practical skills. Following a Red Cross meeting at the Regent Theatre the staff from Namanula volunteered for various tasks and one of my duties was to train the Women's Section of the Rabaul Chinese Emergency Service Company of the Red Cross Society in first aid and home nursing.

News in the Australian papers featured reports every day of the grim war in Europe; in The *Rabaul Times* we read many articles, some of a controversial nature, concerning the role of Japan in world affairs. Over many preceding years the Japanese had systematically invaded and occupied the whole of the north-eastern provinces of China, where heavy concentrations of Military and Naval forces were now being installed. Was Japan planning to penetrate southwards against Indo-China and, perhaps, even the Dutch East Indies?

Japan was, in fact, embarking on a strategy which would threaten the whole Pacific area. The real aim of the Japanese was a southern expansionist programme to create a so-called *New Order in the East* over which Japan would be the dominant force. Japanese Military extremists held powerful sway in the Japanese government; these ex-Samurai were known Fascists and fiercely anti-British. Japan had long ago begun to enforce its *New Order* in China in the guise of *protection of Chinese interests* from foreign control. The Japanese held the wealthiest and most populated cities of the eastern region.

A thorn in the side of Japan was Chiang Kai-shek, leader of the Nationalist Government of China. He could not be persuaded to submit to all Japanese demands; he would not agree to 'peace at any price'. As a consequence Japan formally recognised a *puppet* administration, under Wang Ching-wei (Chiang Kai-shek's long-time rival), as the National Government of the Republic of China.

For quite some time Japan had been encouraged by diplomats of the Axis powers to provoke war. Towards the end of 1940 the Japanese government openly allied with the Axis governments in a Tri-Partite Agreement, which advocated the stabilisation of Europe, Africa and the Far East - *and of Australia*!

Immediately following this Japanese-Axis pact, the United States of America, until now treading neutral ground, allied with the Anti-Aggression powers in recognition of Chiang Kai-shek's regime as the official government of China, thus denouncing the Japanese-sanctioned Wang Ching-wei *puppet* government.

With this phenomenal political development Japan suffered a very serious check in her war-mongering. The American government clearly demonstrated that it did not accept Japan's *Greater East Asia* policy and eventually Japanese-American relations were severed.

In Europe, in 1941, the Second World War was raging. England was being ruthlessly attacked by Germany. North Africa, for the larger part, was on the defensive with the German and Italian Armies mounting attack after attack under the command of General Rommel. The United States of America had not entered the war. In the East, Singapore, with its newly completed Naval Base, was impregnable - Mr Churchill himself had said: "We will hold Singapore no matter what happens". And it was thought, optimistically, that Japan could not really be a great threat to the Pacific.

In Australia, there was much speculation about the worsening political situation surrounding Japan; and most Australians thought that we, in the Territory, were living "too near the Japs for comfort"! In spite of the gloom of that year I enjoyed my first leave home. After being out of touch for so long, it was an exhilarating chapter in my life catching up with friends and family, though getting used to city ways was testing. In relaxed Rabaul, everything in town was within walking distance and shopkeepers were well acquainted with their customers. I had never really lived in a big city, yet Brisbane, revered as just a big country town by its residents, appeared to me to have the hustle and bustle of a thriving metropolis about it. It was almost a welcome relief to depart the city and visit my mother who had moved to Brushgrove in the Northern Rivers District of New South Wales, a beautiful area not unlike the lushness of New Britain.

Some of our friends from Rabaul, who had joined the forces, were training for overseas service near Brisbane and were on leave as well. Among them was Bill Coutts, who was engaged to Joyce. Before he joined up Bill was working for the Bulolo Gold Dredging Company and I had met him on his frequent trips to Rabaul to see Joyce, and even with the never-ending talk of war we all managed to have a happy reunion.

On my return to New Britain I found we had welcomed the arrival in March of the 2/22nd Battalion AIF, known as Lark Force, to protect our shores. An anti-aircraft Battery Unit, under Lieutenant Selby, lent might to the Battalion; an Army hospital was set up by a detachment of Medics from the 2/10th Field Ambulance which included six Army nurses.[3] The troops would have the support of our men of the New Guinea Volunteer Rifles, should the need arise. Later on, in September, the RAAF established a Catalina Squadron in Port Moresby to provide aerial reconnaissance in the South-West Pacific. The squadron was initially equipped with Empire Flying Boats, which

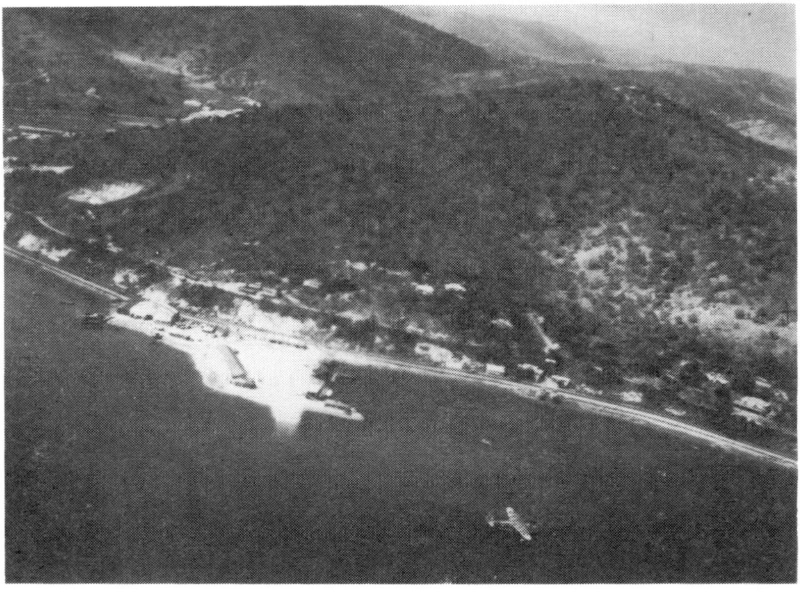

Port Moresby Flying Boat Base

were on charter from the then Qantas Empire Airways, while awaiting delivery of its Catalinas, which could cover a superior range of flight.

Our Matron, Thorbie, was shortly going on leave and on December 8th 1941 she was celebrating with the staff at her farewell party. In shock, we heard the crackling old wireless blare out the Australian Prime Minister's solemn announcement declaring our country to be in a state of war with Japan. This followed the unbelievable and devastating news that the Japanese had bombed the huge American Naval Base in Hawaii. A stunned America retaliated by immediately declaring war on Japan. Three days later two British battleships, *Prince of Wales* and *Repulse*, were dramatically attacked and sunk off the coast of Malaya by Japanese aircraft. How would this effect the impregnable fortress of Singapore, the British Naval base? War had come to the Pacific with surprising rapidity and there was no doubt now of Japan's threat!

Action in Australia was immediate and an Air Force base was established in Rabaul when Number 24 Squadron RAAF, led by Wing Commander Lerew, arrived from Townsville with four Hudson bombers and twelve Australian-built Wirraway aircraft.

The Australian War Cabinet ordered compulsory evacuation

of all European women and children from the Territory and on the 17th of December, when the mail plane arrived, we did not know then that this was to be the last mail we would receive from Australia for many years.

Three days before Christmas the MV *Macdhui* and the *Neptuna* lay waiting in Simpson Harbour to take on evacuees. From the outstations and plantations had come the women and children, the old and sick, missionaries and Government officials. Rabaul had never been called upon to accommodate so many people at one time and was bursting at the seams. Sister Maye, our Administration nurse in Kavieng, brought over her patients, and after a hurried lunch with us departed; we wondered if and when we would see her again.

Against all advice there were a few women who refused to leave their husbands and homes, and among the Methodist missionary community on New Britain four nurses also elected to stay. Doctor Brennan declared government nurses to be in an essential service, but we were given the offer of evacuation if we wished. At Namanula we made our decision to remain, strengthened in the belief that it was our professional duty not to abandon our post in time of certain need.

Amidst the confusion and gloom of this anxious time there were the inevitable lighter moments. Rabaul's comfortable hotels, the Rabaul and Cosmopolitan, overflowed onto the verandahs, and beds appeared in unexpected corners. Many men drowned their sorrows and tried to ease their tension in the peaceful surrounds of the Club. Our popular Chinese cafe, which was usually much frequented by us all, was packed to capacity every evening and in private homes farewell parties went on well into the night.

The day of departure arrived. Down at the harbour embarkation was getting under way when two houseboys, with a pole straddling their shoulders, pushed through the crowd with some last minute laundry: a pair of Madam's corsets and sundry underwear swinging in the breeze. On the heels of these conscientious servants came another. This young man had an outsize toilet seat draped around his neck. It belonged, we were soon told, to a large, jovial lady from one of the islands who declared she'd had this seat made exclusively for her and was not going to Australia without it!

Around dusk the ships finally weighed anchor and the women waved bravely to their menfolk. On the wharf forlorn men in pensive mood watched the safe exodus of their loved ones. Almost all of them would never see one another again.

Rabaul was now a ghost town. Matupi added to the gloom, spraying his almost continual film of grey dust into the air to descend

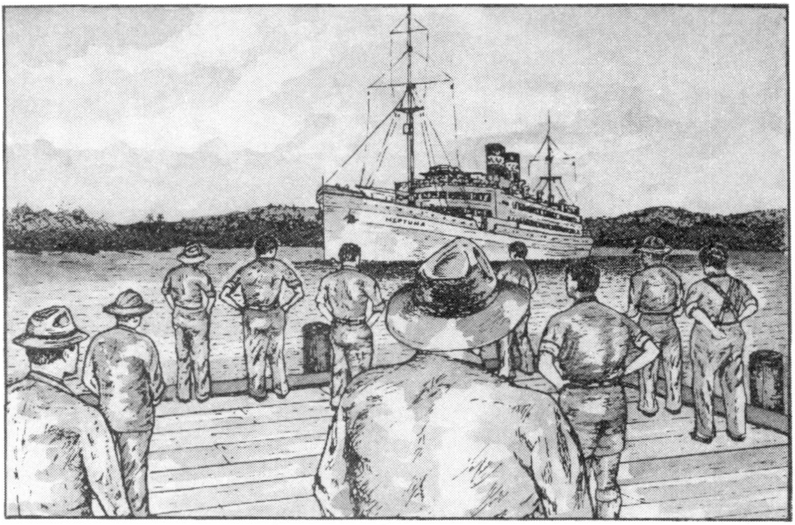

Forlorn men in pensive mood

in a fine mist over the town. Lonely men drifted up the hill to Namanula to chat and have a drink and perhaps a meal, but there was no capturing the spirit of Christmas. Members of the Club, unable to stand the emptiness of their homes, congregated there to talk over old times in a vain attempt to forget their worries.

On Christmas Day the surrender of Hong Kong to the Japanese forces was the prelude to many such events that were to occur at frequent intervals over the coming months.

The festive season was overshadowed by the Japanese threat and celebrations were subdued when Noel and I went to the south coast on Christmas Day to share the occasion with Keith Munro - Heather was now safely in Australia. Here at Kokopo we met the parish priest of Rabaul, Father Barrow, who in the near future was destined to be a great source of help to many of us.

A few days after Christmas the remainder of the women left by plane for Australia, among them was Matron Thorburn. Sister Oldroyd-Harris had come over from Madang just before Christmas Day to take up the position of relieving Matron. Mary Goss, who was a trained nurse, joined us at the hospital and her husband enlisted in the Volunteer Rifles; Mary's husband was a plantation owner and a veteran of the last war. We were now six at Namanula and including the six Army nurses from the Field Ambulance Unit we were the only Australian women left in Rabaul.

A large party gathered at the hospital to usher in the New Year of 1942, but the spirit of hope was missing as apprehension grew daily and the Japanese menace crept nearer. As most of our fears were realised in the months ahead, this year came to be remembered by us and thousands of Australians as the most eventful and tragic year of the Pacific War.

Sunday the 4th January began in the usual lovely way days begin here, with streams of sunshine engulfing the many mountains surrounding us. Mountain climbing in these islands, so close to the Equator, was not very popular with the largely Australian community, nevertheless, during the previous evening at a small dinner party at the hospital, the idea of a climb was suggested. There had been some enthusiasm shown by the men and those of us who would be off duty, yet the only man to arrive this morning among the mountaineers was my friend Noel, and when I called the girls, they too, had a change of mind. Finally, after a very early breakfast and no one else turned up to join us we set out alone.

After climbing for about half an hour the pleasant, rather easy ascent changed. The *kunai* grass was six feet high and its broad, sharp-edged leaves sliced at our bare arms and legs as we struggled upwards, while flies and other insects swarmed around to bite us and buzz at us. We clawed and clambered slowly up the steep, frustrating path and after a final lurch forward reached the top of The Mother. It had taken us two hours to get there and the flat rocky shelf beckoned us to rest and wipe off the blood and sweat of a difficult climb.

The vast scene that lay before us was magic. Blanche Bay, acclaimed as one of the best natural shelters in the South Pacific, stretched to the distance. The sun warmed the cool air and the gentle breeze sent golden ripples across the waters of Simpson Harbour. Island trading schooners dominated smaller craft as they bobbed nonchalantly at anchor. Our two volcanoes, viewed always with guarded uncertainty, presented an even more awesome appearance from here, yet Matupi who had been very troublesome a few weeks ago seemed to respect the peacefulness of the setting and blew his ash out to sea. This of course had more to do with the change in season and a nor' westerly blowing than the spirits of Tavurvur. The giant trees of Malaguna Avenue followed the outline of the harbour, while further inland, the business centre could be seen jutting here and there through the tropical vegetation. Perched on Namanula Hill above the town was the hospital and on the same ridge near by, Government

House. From our lookout on The Mother, we could see clearly why Rabaul could boast one of the most beautiful settings in the islands.

Up there, on top of the mountain, we discussed the war which very recently had seemed so far away. The bombing of Pearl Harbor had jolted the people of the Pacific out of the complacency with which a great many viewed the capability of the Japanese to wage a major war.

In spite of uncertainty of the future, Noel and I set a date to be married at the end of the year when we would be next on leave in Australia and we discussed what, at this stage of the war, could only be an unpredictable future. The sun was now a bright orange-red ball above us heralding a message; it was time to leave the mountain.

'We'll take this path,' Noel said, indicating a narrow opening through the rocks. 'We might avoid some of the *kunai* and ...' We halted, as a loud humming came from high above.

'Must be some of our chaps from Moresby, probably on a reconnaissance trip around the islands. Might be some news for us when we get back.'

Minutes later, a sound as of distant thunder came from the direction of Rabaul and was followed by a spiral of smoke. On this day, 4th January 1942, war came to New Guinea.

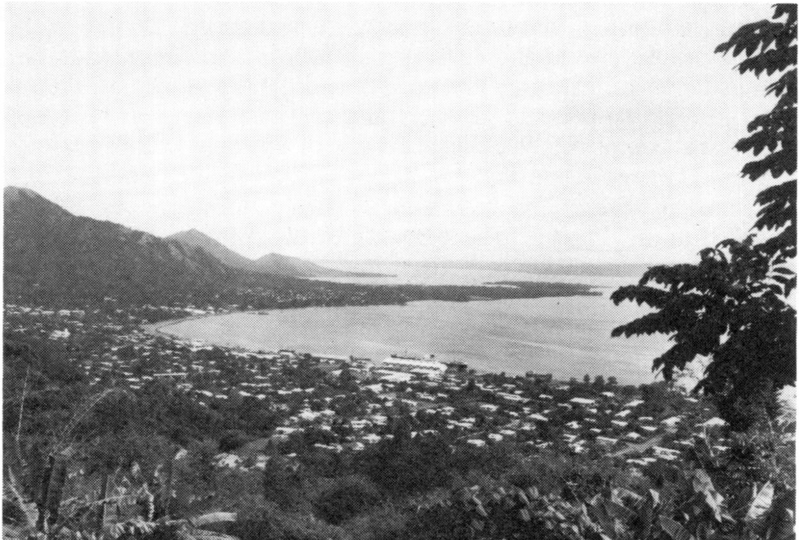

Rabaul

2

RABAUL - WAR

Air raid precautions during the next few days got hastily into full swing; a Red Cross was painted on the roof of Namanula, as well as the Army and native hospitals, and soldiers dug trenches. When the sirens wailed everyone lent a hand in assisting the patients through our maze of paw-paw and banana trees to the protection of the trenches. Like people everywhere we became *blase* after a while and waited until the last minute before leaving for cover. At first many of the alarms were false, but very soon they certainly proved to be the real thing and by necessity we became accustomed to them.

With the constant rain of the tropics, mud in the trenches was an exasperating problem causing among other things frequent changing of uniform. The making of duck-boards stopped us from sinking into the mud and helped protect our shoes somewhat, and we thought khaki overalls might be the answer to our uniform dilemma, accordingly, Joyce and I took a roll of material to the Chinese tailor. Days went by and there was no news of the much needed outfits until one day Angela Choy arrived on duty and made known to us that many of the Chinese community, including the tailor, had *gone bush* while others had taken to the sea and outer islands. Angela was our Chinese sister on the staff at Namanula. Almost daily we were becoming more aware of wartime conditions; and of course we never did get those overalls.

As the raids continued the native staff seemed to sense what was about to happen before the alert sounded. They were always right, and their premature action gave us more time to gather our patients and the necessary equipment before joining them in the trenches.

'Kwiktaim balus (plane) e kom, bombom!' they yelled, heading for shelter early.

These naturally cheerful people took other unusual happenings in their stride as well. One day, in the middle of a raid, our Chinese cook apparently felt he'd had as much as he could stand and joined his companions in the bush leaving the oven full of half-cooked dinner. When his native assistants found the charred contents they proceeded without fuss to *rausim* (throw out) and *kukim kaikai long all*; in other words put on a meal or, as a shearer's cook in the Australian outback would say, "rustle up some tucker for the mob".

The light-hearted disposition of the natives is recounted many times in the tale of most Australian new-comers to the Territory on taking their first swim in these inviting tropical waters. The question asked was always the same.

'Are these waters safe from sharks?'

'Oh, yes, yupela safe,' came the spontaneous reply, 'Im nogat shark hia, im gat only sampela crocodile.'

Late one afternoon the sirens wailed. This was not the usual time for an air raid and anxiety increased as the MV *Malaita*, carrying passengers from the Solomon Islands, entered the harbour. The spirited ship zig-zagged as planes zoomed overhead and our ack-ack guns went into action. When at last the Captain brought his ship alongside the wharf a cheer went up from those on shore and the relieved passengers appeared on deck: planters with their families; traders from outlying islands; and on board as well, Japanese nationals *en route* to internment in Australia!

The *Malaita* was one of the famous seven-letter *M* ships of the thirties belonging to the old Australian shipping and trading company, Burns Philp, well known to all islanders of the South Seas. Captain Wilding, the master of the *Malaita*, was also well known in the islands and regarded as something of a character. He was referred to, with a hint of admiration and perhaps a little envy, as Wild Bill Wilding which gave him a somewhat piratical image: a true 'Master under God'. When some of his crew, understandably perhaps, wanted to leave the ship in Rabaul, he is reported to have issued this ultimatum: "Go ashore and don't come back. Stay with me and I will take you home to Australia".

Serving our area were two aerodromes, Lakunai, close to Rabaul on the flatlands at the foot of Matupi and referred to as the Lower 'drome and Vunakanau, the Upper 'drome, lying inland towards the south. There was severe damage caused to the Upper 'drome with the raid that day. One Wirraway was destroyed and a

Hudson badly damaged, and the almost completed air navigational station received a direct hit. In pursuit of the attacking Japanese Kawanasi flying-boats four Wirraways took to the air and Flight Lieutenant Anderson, at the controls of one of them, gained the distinction of being the first Australian pilot in the Pacific to engage in air to air combat with the enemy.[1]

The following morning saw further destruction to our Squadron when more precious aircraft were destroyed and others damaged in another vicious raid. Bombs fell around the *Malaita* again while still loading at the wharf; however, none found their target and all aboard did arrive safely in Australia, as was the promise of that visionary Shipmaster.

Considering the severity of the bombing there had not been many fatalities, or even many casualties, following the raids. The Japanese were obviously concentrating on the destruction of the aerodromes and essential facilities to create difficulties for our operations, which they effectively did. It was only with the first, totally unexpected raid on the 4th January when the Lower 'drome was hit that, sadly, many natives were killed and many more severely wounded; the slit trenches so quickly, yet efficiently constructed after that protected everyone satisfactorily during the following raids. Our local natives were treated at the native hospital in Rabaul which was competently run by the Administration's Medical Officer, Len Thompson.

When Joyce and I came off morning duty one day we decided to take a look at the aftermath of the bombing. My car was the only one left at the hospital now, the rest had been taken over by the Army.

Near the Upper 'drome we found Wing Commander Lerew ruefully assessing what was left of his damaged quarters which, with the aid of native helpers, had only just been completed. The authorities had stepped in during construction and would allow him to build only one room. The top brass omitted to specify the size, he told us with a wry grin, and that 'one room' had been extended to become a very large, comfortable shack.

'Anyway,' he said philosophically, 'one room or a mansion, it's certainly a well ventilated place now.'

Near by, one of the battered Hudsons was being repaired by its young crew, although to us it looked like something destined for the scrap heap.

'She'll be as good as new in a few hours,' we were assured. 'That's if the Nips leave us alone long enough to get on with the job.' These boys seemed anxious to talk so we stayed for a while with them; we were invited to sit on a plank precariously resting on a couple of oil drums. Others in the Squadron soon gathered round to indulge in casual conversation.

'Anything can happen here,' laughed one of the boys, 'see that tractor over there?' He pointed at the noisy monster working away on the perimeter.

'Well, a few days ago, a native was driving it around during a raid taking no notice of the alert. When he just about got a direct hit, he impulsively made a hasty dive right from the tractor into a trench.'

'That was funny enough,' continued another, 'but when the tractor kept going on without a driver posing a threat to everything in its path we wished we'd had a camera handy.'

'It looked like a scene from a Laurel and Hardy movie,' one of the boys added, and we could picture poor Stanley having to retrieve the runaway tractor, with bombs flying all about, while Olly, in his indomitable style, shouted orders from the security of the trench.

Time being precious to these boys we took our leave and wished them well. We somehow knew they would need all the luck in the world soon; they were to face a mammoth task in the days ahead and some of them would not survive.

Sirens blared alarmingly around noon on the 20th of January and everyone at Namanula and in the vicinity went to the trenches. Almost immediately the familiar hum grew louder and louder as the sky was overcrowded with planes we'd never seen before. Our anti-aircraft guns spat challengingly. The men told us these new-comers were Zero fighters; the personification of Japanese air power. The attack today had an air of insolent confidence about it, as bomber after bomber followed the fighters in endless formation and almost casually dropped their bombs over a wide area around Rabaul. It was estimated that upwards of a hundred planes altogether formed this assault.

Although it was a cloudy day the sky was innocently clear over Lakunai and in stunned disbelief we watched two Wirraways, already in the air on daily patrol duty, engage the enemy with grave results. There were cries of horror and anguish when our six remaining Wirraways appeared and rose to go to certain death in the madness above. These lower powered, trainer aircraft could never match the swift Zero fighter and were virtually powerless against such strength in the number of enemy planes. The odds were further reduced, as six became five, when one of the Wirraways crashed on take-off.

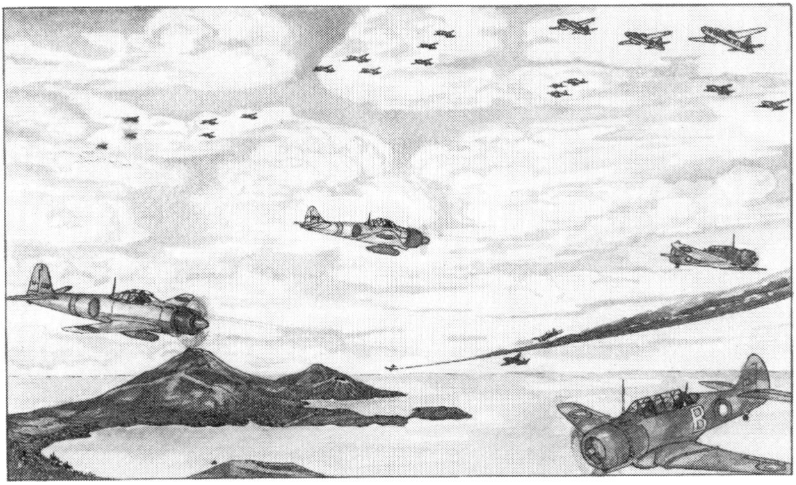

Wirraways courageous, yet impossible challenge

'What the bloody hell are they doing in Australia to have sent these planes here - haven't they learned anything at all about the Japs since Pearl Harbor?' cried one outraged veteran.

The fury of our old soldiers only paused when a crippled Wirraway managed to fire a shot of defiance at a Zero before plunging to earth. The Wirraways and their heroic crews were brought down during this heartbreaking raid, however, two aircraft somehow managed to land safely. With their courageous, yet impossible challenge, a new page of honour was written into Australian wartime history.[2]

When the waterfront became the target the *Herstein*, a Norwegian vessel tied up alongside the wharf, suffered three direct hits and burst into flames. Her daring gunners, firing aggressively at the attacking dive-bombers, valiantly remained at their post until the bridge where the machine gun was positioned collapsed in a wall of flame. The *Herstein* was a defensively equipped merchant ship assigned to the Australian Shipping Control Board in November 1940, not long after Norway's entry into a state of war with Germany. She was delivering ammunition and supplies to bases in New Guinea waters and had arrived in Port Moresby on 3rd January in convoy with the *Aquitania*; the *Aquitania* brought four thousand, five hundred troops to the garrison in Port Moresby.

On delivering her cargo to Rabaul on 14th January the *Herstein* was hoping for a quick turn-round, but was ordered by

Canberra to load a stockpile of several thousand tons of copra - a valued commodity in light of the Japanese advance, and the shortage of shipping, as merchant vessels were requisitioned into the Control Board's shipping pool. With the imminent approach of the Japs, the Deputy Administrator, Harold Page, begged permission of the War Cabinet that the ship be used to evacuate Rabaul's remaining civilians. His urgent plea was not granted and the interpretation of Canberra's response clearly demonstrated that it was a case of *copra* before *people*.[3] The *Herstein* blazed out of control on the 20th January; the wharf and copra sheds quickly caught alight and added to the inferno. The treasured copra was of no value to Australia now!

At last the Japanese turned homewards; our anti-aircraft guns stuttered and a plane broke formation and plunged into the side of The Mother. The only sign of its last resting place was a wing with a vulgar red orb, the insignia of the Rising Sun, standing out incongruously against the tropical vegetation of the mountain.

Soon after the all-clear sounded the ambulance arrived with two wounded in sailor-uniform. The Norwegian sailors had severe burns of the upper body and arms sustained, they told us, when leaving the burning *Herstein*. The operating theatre at Namanula was used by the Army and was the scene of a great deal of tragedy. The Army hospital had been relocated from its unsuitable tent enclosure at Malaguna to Government House, on Namanula Hill. Government House became vacant in November when the Administrator departed as part of the first stage of transferring New Guinea's Administration to Lae. The Army doctors continued to use Namanula's operating theatre as nothing suitable was available at Government House. The natives who had run away to the bush received treatment at the Mission stations around Rabaul. Missions of all denominations were scattered throughout New Britain and the outer islands and they all offered health services to the natives.

Just as the sun was going down a lorry arrived with two of the local volunteers in charge. They gestured towards the vehicle.

'These are the only two we have found so far.'

The battered bodies were almost unrecognisable as the young men we had laughed and joked with a few days ago. One who looked no older than a schoolboy had been shot through the head. The other lay like a discarded puppet, his shattered, broken body had come down in the sea and his partially opened parachute covered him now like a sodden shroud.

News from Australia that evening reported almost casually that Rabaul had again been attacked. There was no mention of the ferocity of the raid, nor of the heroism of the Australian pilots, who faced a formidably superior opponent in the knowledge there was little chance of survival.

Rabaul mourned and buried its dead. The bodies of the Japanese airmen clutching small bags of their country's soil were brought down from the mountain - the first of this enigmatic enemy to be entombed in the soil of this entrusted Territory.

A pall of smoke hovered over Rabaul in the early morning of 21st January and, with a slight breeze blowing, mingled with the smoke from the burning copra sheds and the now drifting hull of the *Herstein* - providing a scenario for the dreadful depression that followed yesterday's bombing. The telephone rang incessantly and there was no end to the advice and speculation given by well-intentioned friends. Many people owned sea-going vessels, some small and some large, and were offering transport south. Others were leaving inland for the south coast in any vehicle that could be coaxed into action. The local natives had almost entirely faded out of sight - mostly on foot - and during the afternoon our friend Keith Munro arrived.

'I've been trying to contact you girls for days,' he said. 'I'm leaving now and ask you to seriously reconsider your position here. We could travel by night. I have made arrangements with friends who left earlier today. We are heading for the south coast where there should be a good chance of being taken out by RAAF flying-boats from Moresby.'

'I will leave you for half an hour,' he said, as we all began talking about the most momentous decision of our lives.

'Start packing,' Keith yelled as he went down the stairs. 'The Japs are coming. They have just about finished their softening-up tactics.'

The vote today was unanimous as it had been a few weeks before when we all agreed to remain. Had we been given a glimpse into the fateful, wasted years ahead that were to seem without end and which benefited no one we would have, I am sure, produced a positive: "We will come with you".

When Keith returned he had his old friend Jimmy Duncan with him. They were surprised and shocked by our decision.

'You think the Japs will observe the Geneva Convention?' Keith said emphatically.

'What about Hong Kong? After landing there on Christmas Day it was reported they plundered and raped until the Emperor of Japan was forced to intervene.'

'Well, if you don't want to chance it with me, Captain Duncan has come with an offer,' Keith encouraged us. 'He'll take you south in the plantation schooner, *Kabakaul*.'

We stood by our decision and gave these good men messages for our relatives and friends in Australia. Keith managed to regain some of his old humour.

'I won't be able to deliver these, Heather will kill me when she hears I left you here.' As they departed an overwhelming sadness descended on all of us.

Later that day volunteers, who had been assisting the demolition squads, arrived at the hospital. After the refugees had taken what they needed for their escape and could carry with them, either by car, schooner or on foot, demolition squads had been busy with the grim work of destroying what might be of use to an invading force.

'We are just waiting around to see what is going to happen next and thought we might be able to give you girls up here a hand.'

These tired men, who were covered with the grime of the morning's destructive operations, were delighted when we invited them to use our showers. Cheerful sounds reverberated from the *haus waswas* as overhead buckets were filled and hauled into position.

'Good of the demolition people not to have wrecked the water pipes along with the power supply,' remarked one of the men as we sat around the tea table later. We were pleased, too, that the hospital had a good stock of that handy emergency stand-by, the primus stove.

We sat talking, discussing anything trivial that came to mind. Before long Oldroyd came over from the hospital.

'A call has just come through from the Health Department,' she said. 'We are to start packing immediately in preparation for evacuation of the hospital.'

There was a moment of stunned silence and then everyone echoed in unison the same question.

'Where will we be going?'

The staff of the Public Health Department had spent a busy time trying to locate anything on wheels in preparation for a quick get away. Strange as it seemed later we had not considered that a move could be pending. We were *greenhorns* and had much to learn about the predicaments of wartime! One of the men suggested that the valley in the hills would be a well-sheltered place to set up a hospital under such urgent circumstances. Apart from somewhere in the bush, no one had any concrete idea as to what form of shelter might be sought.

Members of the Health Department came with papers for the staff to sign. Identity documents were issued stating our role at the hospital and establishing citizenship, and Red Cross arm-bands were distributed, but there was no information about our destination. A phone call to the Army girls confirmed that they were in the same state of suspension as we were with patients ready and waiting to evacuate.

When darkness fell our willing helpers announced that the electricity failure was definitely permanent and we methodically proceeded to haul hurricane lamps out of cupboards and fetch kerosene from the stores. With the aid of the primus stoves and many generous hands a good brew of tea and plates of sandwiches appeared and a picnic-like atmosphere did much to ease the mounting tension.

As the evening wore on guests swelled in number. "Lured by welcoming beacons" one group put it, and for a split second I was transported in time to a memory of yesteryear. The dim kerosene lamp was the only means of light in the vast Australian outback and I had long forgotten its many unsung virtues. Flickering in the darkness of isolated homesteads, it was truly a welcome beacon to lonely swagmen journeying far-reaching horizons in search of work.

Chairs were brought over from the hospital and the present receded for us all as reminiscences took over. A new-comer to the territory asked our colleague from the Health Department how we came to be in possession of all this equipment. And so began again the story of the dramatic eruption of Vulcan Island and its accomplice Matupi.

'When the eruption of '37 occurred the electricity failed, and after things returned to normal,' the officer explained, 'we stocked up with quite a few lamps and stoves for future emergency. Some of them have gone a bit rusty, but most of them work as you can see. One thing is certain though, no one at that time could have possibly envisaged using them for our present crisis. I can tell you I'd gladly swap the Japs' antics for those days, earthquakes, lava and all.' He sounded almost nostalgic and we didn't need to wonder why.

About 10pm Noel came in - I hadn't seen him for days. He was tired and covered in grime as the others had been; he looked as though he'd been fire fighting. After a cold beer from the now dwindling supply our guests brought in earlier today I asked him if he had any plans. As the Government engineer he had been kept busy, over these last weeks, repairing the airstrips after the bombing raids.

'My job is finished now. Today we blew up both 'dromes.'

I told him of Keith's visit that afternoon and of our final decision, which we had discussed earlier.

FORM 13

TERRITORY OF NEW GUINEA

Central Administration,
RABAUL, 12th January, 1942.

I HEREBY CERTIFY that Miss A.M. Bowman, whose signature is appended below, is employed as Nurse, European Hospital in the Department of Public Health.

Deputy Administrator.

Signature:

Australian Government Identity Document

'Well, no one knows what to expect, we can only do what we think is for the best now. The main thing, for the few of us who are staying on, is to stick together whatever happens.'

Doctor Cooper, one of our two doctors, came in around midnight.

'This place is illuminated like Sydney Harbour at Christmas time,' he said in jest. 'The Army camps are blacked out and there are only a few fires burning in the hills.'

After Doctor Cooper greeted our guests and thanked them for their help, he suggested that those who wished to stay could sleep in the empty wards.

'There is the new maternity section too, we are not likely to be needing that for a while.'

Making up beds for these men brought a fleeting sense of normality to this tension filled night; the old patients seemed glad of the diversion and, the added company.

With the coming of dawn a slight breeze blew away some of the murkiness that lingered from the fires and the sun managed to cast a diluted radiance over the sea. There was no joy in this scene. Only a few of our native staff turned up for duty this morning; they instinctively seemed to know when raids were soon to happen. Did they know something dramatic would happen today?

When the sun rose higher, many of the men went off to see what was going on in the town. The five of us of the permanent staff, assisted by Mary Goss and Angela Choy, divided the duties between the wards and the kitchen. Angela, when given the choice to return to her family in the town, had opted to remain with the hospital.

'It will be better here - I knew them in Shanghai!' was her only comment.

'Look im Sister,' yelled the hospital boy who was *brooming* the verandah which overlooked the road leading up from Rabaul. Proceeding slowly up the hill was a column of people; Chinese bearing carts laden with pots and pans, chairs and even a bed; natives followed with head-loads of supplies, food and clothing, dragging their children as they pushed their way onward. This startling spectacle was too much for the orderly, he dropped his broom and with a spring cleared the verandah railing and ran down the hill. When he came back his black eyes were wide with fright and he gestured in the direction of the refugees.

'Im talk liklik taim soldier long Japan e kom.'

When he calmed down a little he told us that the Chinese were fleeing to the nearby valley where a lot of their countrymen had gone already, and the natives, he said, were going to their villages in the bush to the north to escape the anticipated Japanese attack.

The uneasiness on this 22nd of January was almost tangible. The armed forces were noticeably absent from the streets and business centre, and rumours gathered momentum as they spread. The Japanese fleet was said to have left its base at Truk in the Caroline Islands and was headed south. They would by-pass Rabaul, suggested the optimistic, and carry on for an encounter with the Americans in the Pacific. No one as yet had voiced the probability of an invasion of Australia!

'That would be impossible,' was the opinion expressed by those few who were, no doubt, thinking of the last war, but the majority thought otherwise.

'And who the hell is going to stop them!'

New Britain was now undefended in the air. Orders had been received by Wing Commander Lerew to transfer to Port Moresby and form a new squadron. With wounded airmen aboard Squadron Leader Sharp piloted the only remaining aircraft, a Hudson, in a hastily arranged departure shortly before dawn. The balance of the men of Lerew's squadron, whose specialised skills were needed in the RAAF, were ill-equipped to fight. After conferring with the 2/22nd Commander, Lerew led his party - over a hundred in number - on a hazardous evacuation attempt across the island to the south coast, where he hoped to be picked up by flying-boats from the Port Moresby Catalina Squadron.[4]

Under the command of Colonel Scanlan one Australian Battalion, with the support of the dedicated men of the New Guinea Volunteer Rifles, was the totally inadequate resistance available for New Britain. We had neither Navy nor Air Force to assist our small Military force against this enemy of incredible fanaticism and impossible odds. Could defence of an island be achieved without Naval and Air support?

When the alert sounded, our apprehension was tempered with relief in the knowledge that there would be no brave RAAF boys going to face this unrelenting foe in a hopeless attempt to protect Rabaul. As the dreaded hum started, our remaining native staff were already heading for the trenches; those who had *gone bush* after the ominous raid of the 20th had not returned. In the wards Joyce and I were trying to persuade our reluctant, older patients to move to the safety of the trenches also.

'No use going there now Sister,' one veteran was protesting.

'The Japs won't bomb a building of this size,' said another.

'They would have done that earlier, if they weren't so sure they'd be needing it.'

The Norwegian sailors agreed and we all remained in the building.

'I don't know about you,' I said to Joyce as we left the ward for the verandah, 'but my last spark of optimism has just shrivelled up. The old boy is probably right about the reason for leaving this place alone, no other important buildings have been destroyed, have they?'

'Do you think he means that the Japs actually know *what's what* in the town?' Joyce said quietly.

The Japanese Zeros, about forty of them, wheeled and dived like infuriated hawks on their prey as they concentrated on the gun emplacements along the waterfront. Like a delivery of so many parcels and with almost careless abandon the Jap bombers dropped their deadly cargo over the few areas of feeble resistance left. There could be no doubt that this scornful predatory attack was our final softening-up for invasion.

'Where are the bastards going now?' came a shout from one of the crowd gathered on the ward verandah. He was waving a pair of binoculars, and pointing, as bomber followed bomber like a streak of lightning across the sky.

'They're leaving!' someone shouted hopefully. But no one was reassured as the lead bomber headed for the South Daughter.

Concentrating on the Battery at Praed Point, which escaped

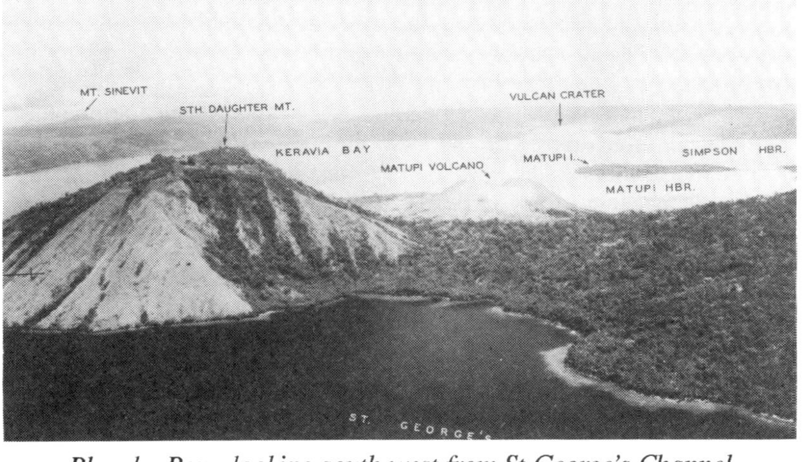

Blanche Bay - looking south-west from St George's Channel

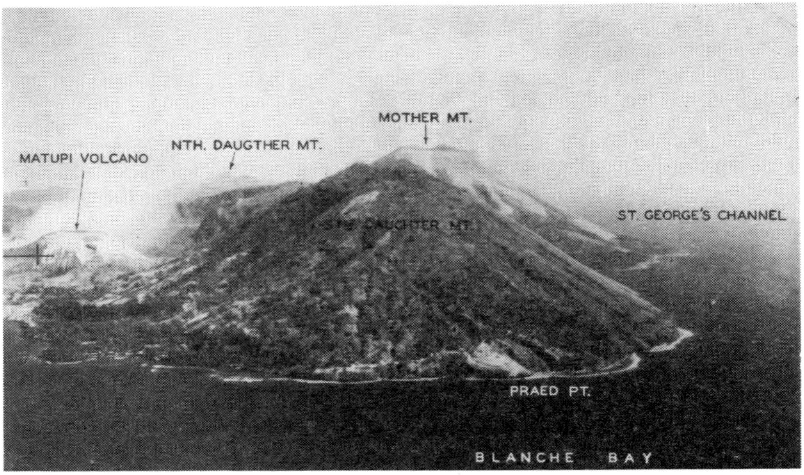

Praed Point Battery - looking north-west from Blanche Bay

the blitz of the 20th, the merciless dive bombers detached a slice of the mountain and sent it hurtling down. The big guns were crushed and tons of rock lay on top of the gallant defenders of our last stronghold. A state of shock overcame the watchers and the agonising quiet was broken by a sombre voice.

'Pray God let those men be dead, when they were buried today.'

'Amen.' Came the response from the silent mourners.[5]

Immediately following the all-clear an invitation was broadcast over the loud speaker: "Help yourselves to everything in the stores before we blow the place up".

Rabaul took on the appearance of a bustling business centre. Grim faced men arrived in the few derelict vehicles that were still around. Customers today wasted no time with friendly greetings and idle chatter as they dragged boxes, bags and any available containers to be filled with essentials for the uncertain days ahead. Chinese arrived with handcarts - there were many who had not fled and still remained in their stores in Chinatown.

Bombs hit the residential area for the first time and the stylish residence of the regional manager of Burns Philp was totally destroyed. The house, only newly constructed, was somewhat of a landmark in Rabaul which vanished when it slipped sideways like a pack of cards and came to rest on a brand new imported car, with all its tyres blown out. Cushions from the lounge lent an absurdly festive air to the trees as their bright coverings fluttered in the sea breeze, however, pieces of iron hurled from the stove added nothing to the decoration of the lawn. A bomb crater, where the swimming pool and coral terraces had once been, completed the pitiful scene.

After the raids the chores of the hospital had always come as a welcome relief, though today our relief was only temporary. Mary Goss was the only experienced housewife among us and proved a great asset as she organised the kitchen staff. Bustling around, our few remaining loyal native boys returned to something like their former selves as they stoked the fire and proceeded to *kukim kaikai long all*. Half way through lunch the phone rang. Oldroyd went to answer it and we all guessed the outcome before she returned, flushed and agitated.

'This is it!' she said.

It was! Doctor Hosking, our Medical Superintendent, and members of the Public Health Department would be arriving almost any minute with all the transport on hand. We were to empty the storerooms and kitchen and get our patients ready immediately.

Assisted by many willing hands the task went smoothly, the bulk packing was already under control with the announcement yesterday. Personal possessions came last in order of priority; transport was limited and we were reduced to one kit-bag each.

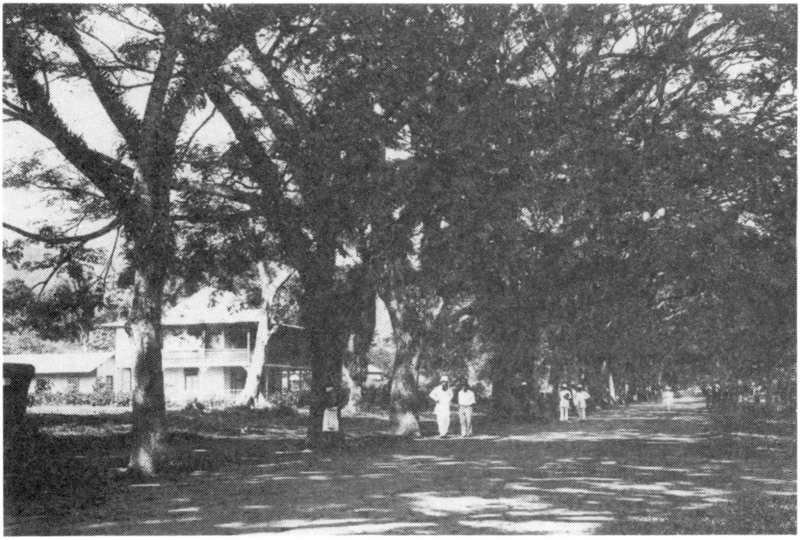

Casuarina Avenue, Rabaul

'The patients and staff will move to the Catholic Mission at Vunapope at once.' This was the order issued by Doctor Hosking on the afternoon of the 22nd January.

'Hurry girls! Cars and trucks are coming to load up now. The Military hospital has already been evacuated.'

Led by the ambulance our convoy came down Namanula Hill skirted the almost deserted town, still hidden in an opaque shroud of smoke, and moved slowly along the once beautiful Malaguna Avenue that framed the harbour with its Casuarina trees. Here, as in Casuarina Avenue in the heart of town, the trees formed a canopy overhead screening the hot tropical sun; now they lay in craters, their giant roots protruding from the mud like monstrous wheels. Anzac House presented a sad sight with its caved-in roof and shattered windows. An Army canteen had been set up at Anzac House, when the 2/22nd arrived almost a year ago, and volunteers from Namanula spent some happy, precious hours giving a helping hand after the women of Rabaul were evacuated last month.

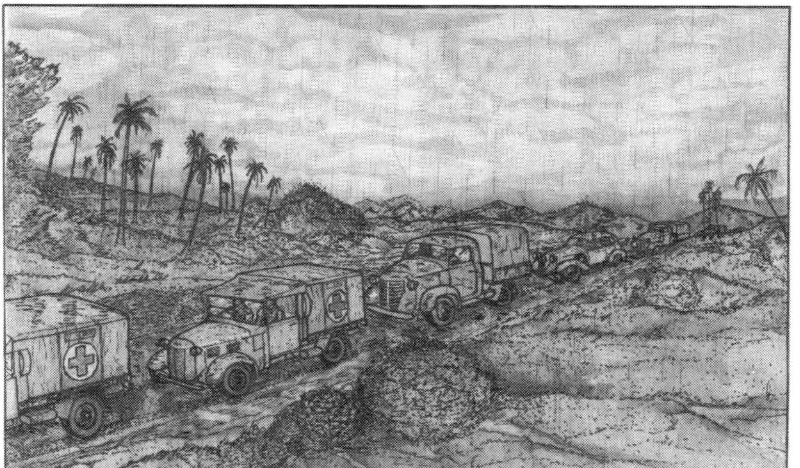

Namanula evacuation convoy

Rain poured down in a deluge to add to the misery. The struggling wheels of the convoy churned up red, muddy water as we splashed through the canyon-like valley beside the naked mound of earth, thrown up by the eruption of '37. This desolate area was dubbed Little Arizona by the men of the 2/22nd, but as our procession of cars and trucks slithered over the slippery, red granite surface it looked more like the Red Sea.

Down on the beachfront could be seen all the paraphernalia of war. Behind miles of rolled barbed wire defences were the once carefree, very young men of Lark Force, tired and strained with the weight of accelerated maturity. Further along, the small contingent of New Guinea Volunteer Rifles was taking up its position. The troops waved and wished us luck as we also waved and wished them luck while crawling slowly past.

Standing beside their guns in readiness for the colossal task ahead, it was difficult to hold the memory of all these men as the happy men we had known. The recent bombing raids had turned the Japanese menace from a vague and distant threat to one that had suddenly come alive like a venomous snake emerging from under the grass, to strike.

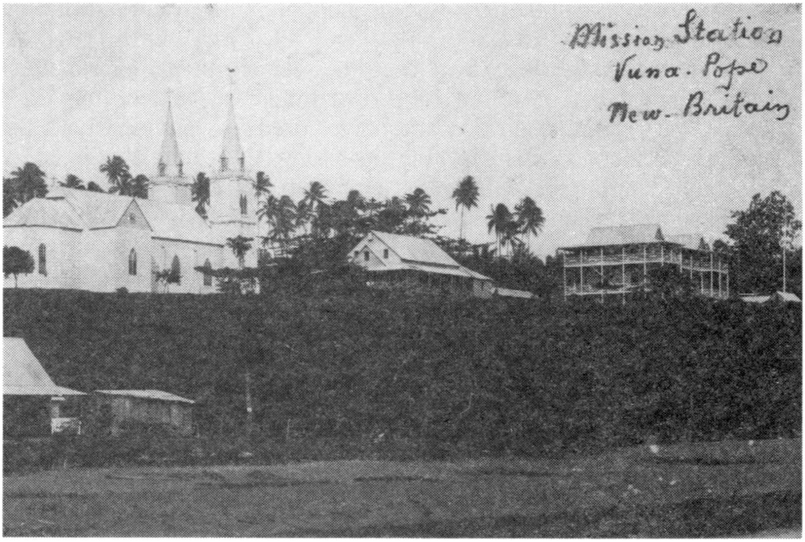

The Sacred Heart Mission, Vunapope (early 1900s)

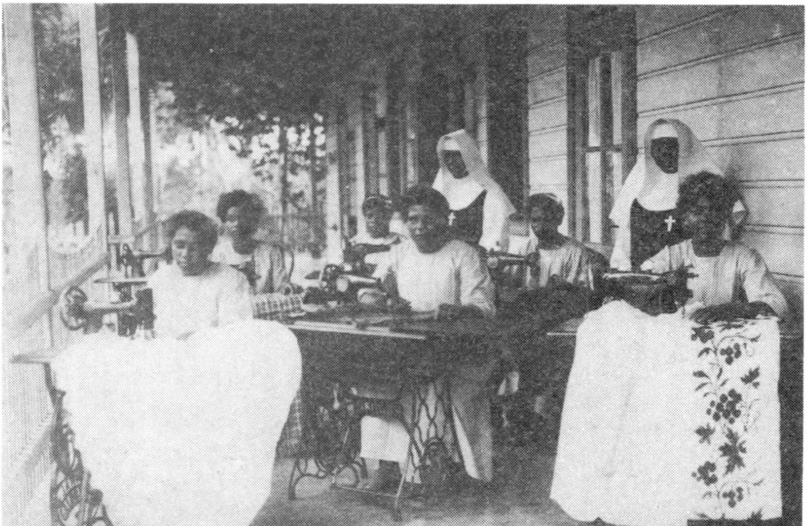

Native Girls' Boarding School - Administration Hospital

3

VUNAPOPE - REFUGE

As we approached Vunapope the rain eased somewhat and a mellowing sun caught the glistening spires of the cathedral concealed among the trees and settled misty shafts of light on the scene that unfolded before us. Solid white buildings, divided by lush green lawns and gravel paths of white coral, lay spread out like a painting on a canvas. We had arrived at the Mission.

Our convoy came to a halt and small native boys wearing Red Cross armbands directed the drivers to a large two-storey building, which was one of the Mission's native boarding schools and had been hurriedly converted for our use. In the dormitory, which was on the ground floor, beds were prepared and cupboards made available for storage. Furnished with tables and chairs, the wide verandah provided a very comfortable relaxation area. Closer inspection of a nearby building revealed convenient washing and toilet facilities.

The men unloaded our packing cases and stacked them on the verandah. With the help of the Doctors we unpacked the cases and sorted out medical supplies before putting them into the cupboards. The obvious organisation and thoughtfulness that prevailed here was like a balm on strained nerves and the last few chaotic weeks receded into the background. Our patients were settled without fuss into a ward where all was in readiness to receive them.

About an hour later the heavy work had come to an end; it was time to think about food and how we would manage preparation in that department.

Rather wearily, Joyce and I started sorting out various tinned stock and the few fresh vegetables we were able to pack when over the lawns came two natives in white uniforms. Hanging from a pole across their shoulders was a very large, covered cooking-pot swinging rhythmically between them as they paced along. What a relief to see the evening meal.

We had never tasted a stew such as this before. There was an undefinable flavour of herbs and spices about it missing from Australian cooking of pre-war days, except among continental people, and we all agreed that hospital cooking was *never like this*. In the hungry years ahead we were to take a nostalgic look back, many times, at this particular evening and the nuns' stew.

The abrupt change from our last days in Rabaul to the tranquillity of Vunapope was so unbelievable as to make the present seem unreal.

'Don't let's talk about Japs and bombs, let's savour the peace of this evening,' Grace said as we joined a group relaxing on the open verandah. Grace wanted to banish anxiety from her mind and allow her thoughts to go back to her native Townsville.

Sitting among the palms in the security of the Mission, it was easy to drift in time to those idyllic tropical places on the far north coast of Queensland, such places as Townsville, Cairns, Magnetic Island, holding special memories. The end of the day all over the tropics is the most pleasant time, when the humid air dissipates with the gentle evening breeze. At Vunapope the air was flower scented and free of smoke; we basked in the fragrant serenity, and even the mosquitos seemed to be singing as they stung us kindly.

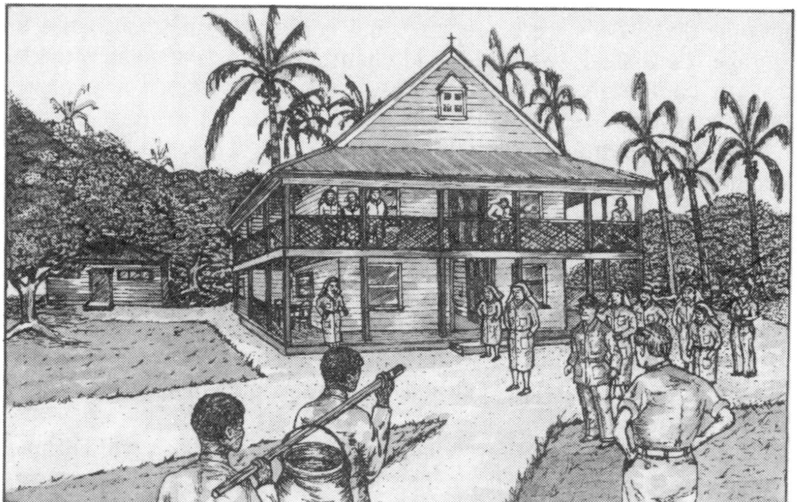

The evening meal

'The mosquitoes are kept to a minimum by proper control of the environment, no doubt.' This comment by one of the more scientifically minded men jolted us back to reality.

Dusk came quickly and the Angelus-bell rang out. A short time later two nuns came towards us from the direction of the Chapel.

'We hope you are comfortable,' they said as we rose to meet them. These Australian Sisters stayed a short while with us and, on leaving, promised to return in the morning.

'Sleep well and peacefully tonight, and God bless.'

'Thank you Sisters,' one of the men called out, 'only an earthquake will keep us awake tonight.' He couldn't have been more wrong - only the unconscious or the dead were to sleep that night!

The men asked us to choose our sleeping area and we settled on the open verandah upstairs where a cool breeze was being fanned in from the sea. We voted the canvas stretchers surprisingly comfortable, but no complaints would have come forth this evening had our resting place been a slab of concrete. It had been an exhausting day and as the gentle rain made tapping noises on the iron roof it blended harmoniously with blissful thoughts of a long, relaxing sleep.

The first to give the alarm were the veterans who were sleeping in a nearby room. A battle was raging just a few miles along the coast and we felt as though we were *there* as the old soldiers, in turn, took over the role of commentator.

'Rabaul is being attacked; they're shelling the place.' 'The bastards are trying to land!' 'Jap ships are giving cover.' 'God help our boys up there.'

We wondered if the Japs knew how small the contingent was out there defending the beachfront. We, who had waved and wished them luck such a short time ago as they stood with their guns behind the barbed wire on the beach, were faced with the grim fact that their hour had now come. The last two raids had demonstrated the potent ferocity of the Japanese and the odds would be strongly stacked against our men. Pearl Harbor and Hong Kong left no doubt in the minds of anyone that an invasion by Japan would not mean, at least, supremacy in number.

'We know the Aussies are tied up in North Africa and Europe, but the Yanks are supposed to be in Moresby and must be just rearing to have a go at these Nip bastards.'

The rhythm changed now as explosions added to the din.

'Those are mortars - the Japs must be coming ashore and our boys are throwing mortars into the barges.'

As star-shaped lights lit the sky and burst into sprays the scene took on the appearance of a Guy Fawkes night fireworks display.

'Those are coming from the Jap ships.'

Bold rat-tatting of machine guns could be heard in futile defiance. The sky over Rabaul was illuminated to daylight brightness as low-flying planes began dropping flares. At intervals during this endless night the primus was lit downstairs and tea made. Discussions began again about the possible behaviour of the Japs who were now on our doorstep, though no one could add anything to our previous deliberations.

When the filtered golden glow of dawn dutifully began to break the battle waned, but there was no comfort in the comments from the veterans.

'I'm afraid the Japs have landed.' 'God be with our boys and everyone else.'

We proceeded in apprehensive silence to the waterfront at Vunapope where we found many of the missionaries.

The sight that met our eyes was mind-boggling. Stretched as far as the eye could see were ships of every size and description: frigates, freighters, tankers, transports and barges.

The fleet was moving slowly and silently around Praed Point at the tip of the peninsula to join others already anchored at the foot of Rabaul; and on the horizon two huge aircraft carriers stood like

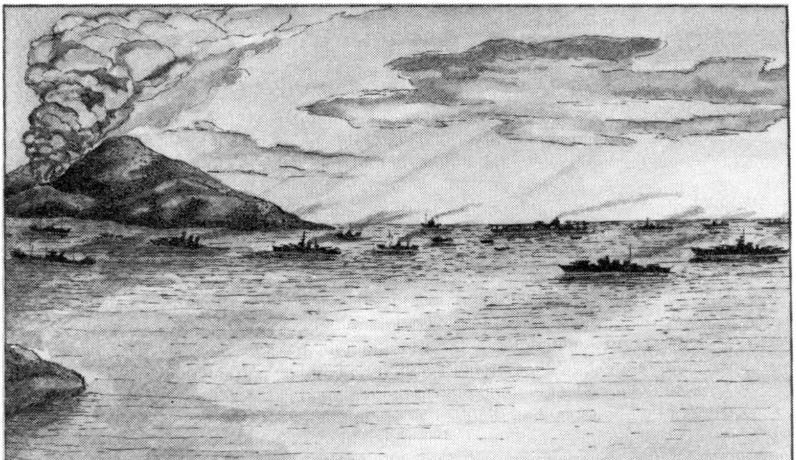

The Japanese Imperial Navy

sentinels. The wrath of the waves breaking on the shore was all that could be heard. The watchers stood mesmerised in stunned disbelief by this terrible spectacle - the final evidence that the enemy had indeed landed and was now in control of this island of New Britain.

The silence was broken by the Mission bell ringing for first mass.

'Come now,' said an Australian nun, 'we must pray, let us go to the chapel.' We followed her like a group of obedient school children.

The missionaries, with their trained and dedicated minds, were probably the only ones giving full attention to the service this morning. We were hearing the shock of distant explosions intermingling at intervals with the unnerving whirr of planes overhead. We, the newcomers, were jolted out of our mixed emotions when the priest made the announcement that we must pray for the one in our community who gave birth to a baby girl early this morning. The baby's father was the Mission's doctor who came with his wife from Germany some years ago.

Germans! The thought immediately crossed my mind that if these people were Germans the Japs would surely treat them favourably. We walked somewhat dazed from the chapel and Joyce showed her compassionate nature when we discussed the untimely birth of that baby.[1]

'I can't help thinking of that poor woman with a new baby and we think we've got troubles.'

After mass one of our men handed us a sheet of paper.

'I just got this over my radio and it is hard to believe.' We all agreed with his statement as we crowded around and heard him read the message.

'No news from Rabaul since 4pm yesterday, there is no truth, whatsoever, that the Japanese Navy has entered Rabaul Harbour.'

'What on earth is going on down there?' someone asked as if calling for an answer.

'Where are their planes that they can't come over and see what's happening here? After all, we're not that far away and if their reconnaissance is this bad the Nips will have Aussie while they're asleep!' Various comments from the men were expressed, while worries about parents, relatives and friends, who by now must have fears mixed with confusion for our safety, remained unspoken.

'Look, here they come!' Noel exclaimed. There was a roar of engines as two Jap Zeros flew so low they skimmed the tree tops near the cathedral; from under the wings orange-red orbs glared like grotesque eyes. As the aircraft continued to circle over the Mission the hypnotic effect was finally broken when a voice called out loudly.

'Just like a bloody hawk having a good look at its prey.'

We were relieved, to say the least, to watch them fly away and the groups under the coconut palms wandered off to their quarters. Two of our girls had come back earlier and already had the primus working. Never had tea been so appreciated!

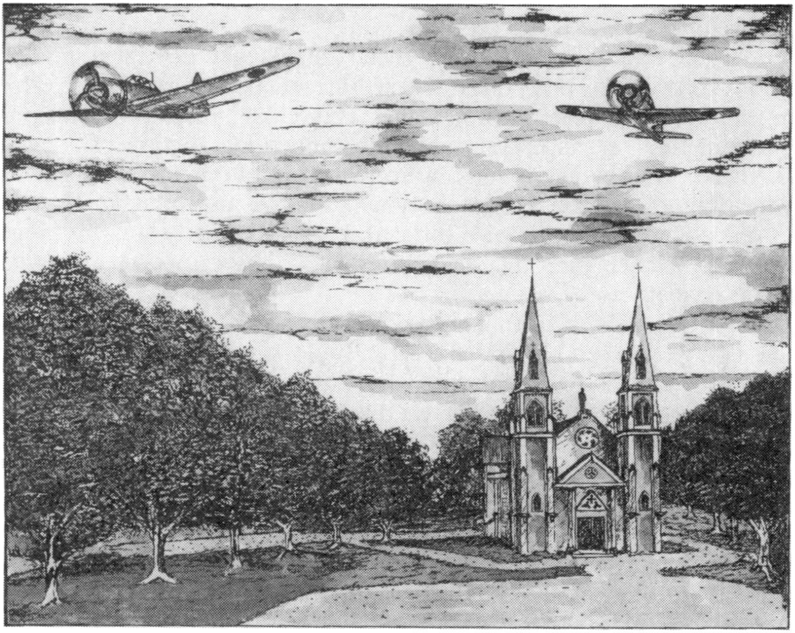

Zeros over the Cathedral

The beauty of our first morning at this welcome retreat could not be enjoyed. It was one of those fresh tropical mornings with the distinctive bouquet from overladen Frangipani trees wafting, as always, all around in the cool breeze and here at Vunapope the aroma stifled the gentle fragrance of the nuns' flower gardens. In spite of this, tension hung over everything like a thick fog and a strange weightlessness filled the empty vacuum within us. It was as though a great tiredness had fallen over us and there was nothing to do or say - just wait!

As the sun rose higher over the bay there was no conversation among the crowd gathered on the upstairs verandah of the building allotted to us. Almost the only sound came from the drone of distant aircraft and blasts from tugs chuffing around the Japanese ships manoeuvring in the harbour.

With frightening majesty, ship continued to follow ship into the channel, passed the sentinels of Vulcan and Matupi, to come to rest in Simpson Harbour under the questioning eye of The Mother. A terrible fascination for the scene being enacted in the bay drew us forward again and again to watch. On this fatal day even nature was in league with the enemy as the wind caught the grey ash from Matupi's crater and swirled it away from Rabaul. With aching hearts we witnessed the solemn intrusion of the Japanese Imperial Navy on that morning of the 23rd day of January 1942, and our fate was sealed.

'I suppose it's too much to expect that these bloody Japs will treat our boys like we treated our Germans back in 1914, when we took this island from them.' One old-timer was reminiscing.

A hush seemed to hang over the ships now sheltered in the harbour. As this indescribable morning wore on rumours began to circulate, true or false no one really knew. No news had come over the radio from Australia since early that morning. Around noon messages came through to Vunapope that the Australians were in retreat and that the Commander had given the order "Every man for himself".

This, then, was the end of the campaign for the heroic defenders of Rabaul. What of the fate of survivors? There had been no preparation for withdrawal. In fact the Australian Government had said there shall be no withdrawal! Most of the soldiers would have absolutely no knowledge of tropical bushcraft, essential, if they were to become engaged in guerilla warfare or seek escape via the jungle to the other side of the island and get away by sea.

This was a very anxious time for Mary. Her husband Tom was one of the New Guinea Volunteer Rifles stalwarts, whose vital role was among those in the first line of defence on the beach. Having served in the First World War he was well experienced and we sincerely believed he would have survived the battle. We did our best to allay Mary's fears. Tom Goss was a planter who knew the island well and could speak the local language, advantages in favour of any quest for escape.

Meanwhile, at Vunapope, the missionaries had already gone into the bush they knew so well to seek out refugees and give whatever assistance might be needed. Early in the afternoon they brought in three very shell-shocked young soldiers to the ward and then went off again to continue their search. In the days and weeks that followed, these good Samaritans were to persevere with their rescue work giving comfort and refuge to the soldiers, civilians and natives who had been caught up in the aftermath of invasion and were ill-equipped for the ordeal ahead of them. Many were to succumb very quickly to the scourges of dysentery and malaria accompanying harsh living in the inhospitable jungle. In this climate a minor scratch, if not effectively treated, could turn with incredible haste to a frightful tropical ulcer with debilitating results. Malnutrition and starvation would soon affront them.

That afternoon exclamations of astonishment from the men sitting outside brought us all to our feet. The shrubs on the borders of the garden seemed to be moving and from them emerged small figures resembling leaf-covered monkeys carrying outsize handkerchiefs. After staring at us for a short time they spread the brightly coloured cloths on the ground and proceeded to strip the trees of mangoes, paw-paws and bananas, and while so doing shed most of their camouflage to reveal khaki caps and uniforms.

'Well, I'll be damned!' I heard one of the men exclaim. 'Who would believe that our first sight of the enemy would be a gang in the guise of school boys pinching fruit?'

Yet more Japs, draped in the camouflage of net and twigs, visited us during that afternoon. They just stood and stared without speaking.

'Maybe we are the first Europeans they have ever seen, the Japs in this bunch look like a group of country boys to me,' one of the men commented.

'Just a troop of monkeys on their way back to the trees,' added another.

On this ill-fated day Rabaul had surrendered to an invasion force of many thousands. The Australians, an Army of one thousand four hundred men - hopelessly outnumbered - held out for ten long hours. At dawn they had seen the Japanese pile their dead on the rolled barbed wire on the beach; the invaders made a landing over a bridge of their dead comrades.

No further casualties had come into the wards at either of the hospitals - the missionaries had set aside the sixty-bed Mission hospital for the Army nurses. For us, the day was filled with suspense, and there was no relief in sight. As the sun set an eerie calm hung over Vunapope where suspense reigned supreme. Japan's victories, one after the other, had been achieved with such incredible swiftness in the short period since Pearl Harbor that little was known about the fate of people captured and we had no idea what to expect.

Later in the evening Joyce produced a special bottle of champagne she had been saving. Noel and Doctor Cooper joined us on the lawn; these two had been ardent competitors in the Rifle Club and were good friends. They had won many trophies over the years as both were top scorers for their teams - Noel, the Public Works Department and Doctor Cooper, the Health Department. How peaceful everything seemed and the enemy only a few miles away!

The next day more men who had fought in the battle were forced, through exhaustion and their wounds, to rest in the bush and those unable to continue were brought in by the missionaries. The worst cases were admitted to the ward and the others joined a rapidly increasing community upstairs. One of the brothers told us later that those who had already been picked up by flying-boat on the south coast are to be considered among the fortunate. By reports received there were some who had been rescued and Joyce and I hoped that Keith Munro and his friends were among them. With the passing of every day chances of rescue would be even more hazardous. Patrols were penetrating the island inland and when the Japanese turn their attention to the southern coastal areas the seas would be swarming with shipping, making rescue by flying-boat impossible.

'We can only pray for them - and quickly find as many as possible,' the Brother said.

Low-flying planes buzzed around the skies and ships again manoeuvred in the harbour for suitable moorings to off-load equipment and supplies. The day was alive with movement. Around the Mission small groups of Jap soldiers continued to raid fruit trees while others lingered, to stand and stare at us - they seemed as uncertain of us as we were of them. Many of these intruders rode in on bicycles, having no doubt taken them from their native owners.

There had been a lot of supposition which produced very little optimism when the sun set on the evening of January the 24th. We experienced another exhausting day of tension and unreality, not knowing, yet wondering what the Japs might do.

Almost forty-eight hours had passed since the invasion and the brief twilight was darkening when we heard the sound of vehicles crunching to a halt on the gravel drive. Japanese soldiers jumped from them and four heavily braided officers, with long swords clinking, came towards the verandah. Guards stood at attention as two of the officers ran up the stairs. One officer shouted at a guard and pointed to us while the other gave his attention to the men in the group.

The seven of us were herded downstairs and lined up some distance from the building. The men were given similar treatment not far away and it was amazing how their presence gave us reassurance. When the Jap officer shouted a command in perfect English our immediate response registered shock; whispering ceased instantly.

'Hands above your heads and keep them there.'

Two of the officers made a quick search of us by running their hands down our uniforms and ending up, for some reason, stroking their fingers through our hair. Angela Choy, standing beside me, came in for special attention.

'Shina!' shouted the officer as he flashed a torch in her face; thankfully, without further comment he moved on.

We must have been left standing for at least an hour - it was pitch dark now; the officers had disappeared and the Japs guarding us seemed detached and bored.

'I think I can hear our men talking somewhere over there,' I plucked up the courage to whisper to Joyce. The men were nowhere in sight and obviously far from us, but we had begun to relax a little.

Very quietly, one of the officers returned with orders for the guard, who yelled at us in Japanese and hustled us off with a wave of his rifle.

'Hayaku (quickly)!'

We came onto a verandah. More guards joined the procession and flung open the door of a narrow storage room at the rear of the building. Several of our patients were in here sitting against the wall on the concrete floor. The guard closed the door and to our horror we heard the key turn in the lock. The room had no windows and the only vent for air was the space between the door and the floor.

To everyone's great surprise there was another elderly man with the patients whom we recognised as Doctor Watch. Doctor Watch was originally from South Africa and had been in private practice in Rabaul for many years. He was not a young man and we'd naturally assumed he had gone to Australia with the evacuees last month; he was as amazed to see us here as we were to see him. After a preliminary exchange of news he told us that the Japanese had brought him here from his home in Rabaul. The other civilians in the town who had not sought escape, together with the soldiers, were rounded up and confined in the 2/22nd's Malaguna Road camp.

'I expect them to adhere to the rules of the Geneva Convention,' he said, 'as was done in the last war.' Doctor Watch was a veteran of that war and had served in France. Did he really believe what he'd said or did he make the statement for our benefit?

We noticed the three soldiers suffering from shell-shock huddled together at the end of the room.

'I spoke to them just after the Japs brought them in here,' the Doctor said, 'but I couldn't do much to help them. Those blasted Japs took everything from me before I left my house and promised, when I made a fuss, that my medical bag would be returned to me later.'

Distant explosions shook the building at intervals and in the darkness of this almost airless room there was only whispered conversation and wishful thinking overshadowed with anxiety. Perhaps help from Moresby was at hand, from the sounds ringing out the Cat-boats, as the men called our Catalinas from the Port Moresby squadron, were causing damage somewhere near with their accurate bombing. The young soldiers had dropped into an exhausted sleep and it seemed nothing could possibly disturb them.

Towards midnight the lights came on and the door was flung open by a Japanese officer. To our amazement he approached Doctor Watch and proceeded to shake him by the hand.

'I have good news,' he said. 'We are now friends. The Japanese Imperial Navy is in control of the Pacific and will proceed to Australia. Peace has been declared.'

'Bloody ridiculous,' muttered Doctor Watch, as he rose slowly from the floor. 'The fellow must be drunk.'

This last statement was no doubt true. The Japanese officer ignored the women prisoners and staggered over to the patients. However, before he was able to make any announcement the soldier, who had suffered the most from shock, leapt to his feet and exploded in a torrent of mad abuse. When the Jap put his hand to his sword we watched frozen with horror. For a suspense-filled moment he paused, and after what seemed a split-second decision turned and swayed towards the door. None of us, witnessing this irrational action on the part of the distressed soldier, and the Jap officer's considered reaction, realised that the Japanese have a superstitious horror of mental aberrations, even of a temporary nature.

There was one observation we did make which clearly stood out and left us more than a little bewildered. The Japanese officers enjoyed a reasonable command of the English language. Could this have been part of the broad plan to loot with greater ease the Colonies of the British Empire?

'You girls should never have been left here,' Doctor Watch said. He was rather breathless now as he eased himself down onto the concrete.

'And I am beginning to think I am a fool too, to do this again at my age.'[2]

This dreadful night wore on as if it would never end. In the early hours of the morning four half drunken Japs flung the door open and beckoned to four of us women to come outside. "Too much hot in here" one seemed to mutter. When completely ignored he hesitated, trying to dredge up more English, but "Make tea" was clearly understood. When ignored again, one of his pals aimed a punch at my head which I just managed to dodge. Suddenly, footsteps were heard outside and this quartet became excited and made a hasty exit. No one at this stage spoke of the terror the visit aroused.

'I'm just glad the boys there didn't wake up,' came Joyce's hushed comment to me.

The visits by the Japs that night had one advantage - the fresh air that came in with them. The effect of distant explosions and dreams of rescue by the Americans faded as the night progressed and the more pressing problem of lack of air and high humidity gained top priority. The only ones enjoying respite were the soldiers brought in from the bush that day; they slept the sleep of sheer exhaustion.

Doctor Watch had no information as to the whereabouts of our men and thoughts of their fate left our minds only when we began to wonder about the confusing reports our families would probably be receiving if news from Rabaul really had not got through to Australia as was reported yesterday.

'I was driven to Vunapope and put straight into this room,' said Doctor Watch. 'As far as I could make out I was the sole occupant of the building before they brought the patients in.'

We asked Doctor Watch if he knew whether it was true or not that no news had been received of Rabaul in Australia. He told us that he was sure that communications would have been established by teleradio, and Port Moresby would have received news. Apparently confusion arose when the disposal team set off a bomb dump along the Malaguna roadside on the afternoon of the 22nd. The radio transmitter at headquarters was put out of action, as were all the valves in all the radio sets in the town, when the bombs exploded. Ironically, these were the many tons of bombs, which were requested by Wing Commander Lerew and had just been discharged from the ill-fated *Herstein* only a few days previous.

The clatter of crockery in the early morning transferred our worries to another subject and it was something of a relief to have this trivial distraction. What was happening to our supplies of tea and sugar? And had everything been locked away as Oldroyd suggested?

'Don't worry,' Lik said, 'the Japs only drink green tea - I could do with a good strong cup now, the real thing I mean.'

Like nurses everywhere we were labelled with nicknames or

simply referred to by our surnames. Jean McLellan was very small of build and was called Lik, from the Pidgin *liklik* meaning little. As an exception to this rule I always called Joyce by her given name, whereas the others called her Mac; I, on the other hand, have always been called Bowie.

With the welcome approach of dawn breathing had become increasingly difficult in this almost sealed room and Doctor Watch was showing signs of restlessness. Suddenly the door was flung open again. Fortunately the soldiers continued to sleep undisturbed, but we were startled and tried not to show our frayed nerves by feigning sleep, hoping to be ignored. The Jap before us was carrying a box which he placed in the doorway. He squatted on the box facing to the outside and was obviously on guard duty. He was hardly a reassuring sight silhouetted in the frame of the open door with his rifle and fixed bayonet ready for action, but a slight breeze was stirring now and the cool, sweet air coming in was like a gift from heaven.

Sometime after sunrise we heard a clumping of boots outside and a high pitched voice called out something which sounded like *Tenko* - this was a word that was to become so familiar to us we were never to forget it for the rest of our lives. *Tenko* is the Japanese name for roll-call with, sometimes, its own special zest. We were taken outside and put into line to be painstakingly counted by the 'night watch'. After a few comments, several bows were exchanged between the two guards before our night guard marched off duty with his colleagues. This day-duty guard was very young and looked indecisive. He stood with a fixed look for a few breath-holding seconds and then casually ambled some distance away, and together we breathed audible sighs of relief when allowed to disperse.

More relaxed now we set to and started gathering up the scattered, but mostly intact, crockery. We almost dropped it ourselves when we heard the sound of men's voices coming from around the corner at the other end of the building. The relief at seeing one another was mutual. The men appeared in comparatively good spirits as we exchanged news of our first night as prisoners of war.

'Anyway, you girls are *okay* that's the main thing. Now what's for breakfast?' Leaving us with this query they went off to the ablution rooms. Their guard joined ours and we began preparing breakfast for the patients, the men and ourselves. Oldroyd went with the doctors to see the patients under our care; most of them had remained in the ward during the night.

We were soon interrupted in our domestic duties by two Japanese who arrived dragging sacks which they emptied out in front of us. We noticed the Australian brands on the tins of fish scattered over the kitchen floor - the invaders had lost no time in helping themselves to the goods of the conquered. The Japs pointed to the loaves of bread and indicated that they were to be sliced, and *make tea*. Though these two words seemed to come easily to the guards, by this time we had discovered that they, quite definitely, did not enjoy a command of the English language. When the men who had joined us again tried to help with this chore, by attempting to light the primus, one of the guards made a barrier with his rifle - preparation of food was for women only.

Two more Japanese arrived on the scene carrying bundles from which they produced cooked rice, bowls and chopsticks.

'This lot are really making themselves at home,' I said to Mary as they proceeded to lay the items on stools, brought out from the rooms. We were about to be initiated into the eating habits of the Japanese and not one of us was prepared for the ensuing phenomena. The unwelcome guests squatted on the floor and, with bowl of rice at mouth level, literally shovelled in large quantities, interspersed with many grunts and much belching.

'Makes me feel homesick,' Joyce whispered. 'Just like the pigs on the farm.'

Joyce was quite familiar with the habits of these fat little, four-legged animals. She came from a farming property at the foot of majestic Mount Sturt near Warwick on the rich pasture lands of the Darling Downs. Joyce's forebears were pioneers of that well-known area in Queensland. The Japs wiped their mouths on the sleeves of their uniforms when the meal was over. They put their unwashed bowls and chopsticks back into bundles and indicated that we might eat as, without ceremony, they took their leave.

'So much for male Japanese manners, I wonder if the women gobble up food like that too,' remarked one of the men.

There was almost a feeling of light-heartedness in the way everyone lent a hand with preparing our own breakfast, no doubt due to the departure of the Jap guards and the easing of tension of these last twelve, uncertain hours since the Japs made their appearance at the Mission. A large tub of porridge arrived from the Mission kitchen and lightened the catering work considerably. To a distant observer we could have been taken for a carefree crowd as we sat on the lawn after the meal drinking tea. The thought was comforting even if only for the brief moment; we were still unsure what to expect from the Japs.

Many of the older men kept falling asleep as the morning

wore on and it was then that we heard what really had happened to them the previous night. Two guards had taken them into a large room in one of the Mission out-buildings and made them sit on the hard concrete floor. They were to remain with their knees tucked under their chins and hands flat on the floor and told, that should there be the slightest movement from any one of them, they would all be shot. The guards kept a machine gun trained on them all night! After listening to this harrowing story we appreciated all the more the fact that, in comparison, we had 'got off lightly'.

The nursing staff left the men to rest. After attending to patients and making beds we decided to go upstairs, where we had all slept on our first night, and retrieve some of our property left there.

Napoleon is supposed to have said, that a sure sign of victory is to sleep in the beds of the conquered. An all-night orgy must have wiled away the hours for these conquering heroes, though perhaps not in the way the hero of the French had in mind. Mosquito nets lay in a tangled mess on the floor, some of our canvas stretchers were smashed and thrown aside, bayoneted food tins were strewn everywhere and the contents trampled into the sheets.

Stepping warily between broken bottles and jagged tins we searched for the few prized possessions, mostly of sentimental value, that we were able to bring with us. Many of them were missing and others damaged beyond repair. In subdued silence, as if controlled by a mysterious force, we cleaned the mess and swept away the debris.

'I think we must make up our minds that we are prisoners of war now,' Grace said, 'for the time being anyway.'

The next few days left no doubt in anyone's mind into which category we belonged.

Later in the morning in a period of quiet the Sisters from the Army hospital appeared. They were accommodated in the Dutch precinct of the Mission. They said they had spent a comparatively trouble free night and went on to tell us that they too had Jap visitors this morning.

Apparently two Japanese privates arrived as they were giving the patients breakfast. Whytie (Lorna Whyte) described this pair as looking like a cross between *beings* from outer space and monkeys, who jabbered shrilly and proceeded to make themselves objectionable. Whytie was the youngest of the Army girls, in fact the youngest of us all, and was never shy to speak her mind. They snatched food from the patients, she said, and threw it on the floor and refused to let the Sisters near their charges.

When the Japs tired of trying to provoke the men they tried

out their English on Cal (Eileen Callaghan), who ignored them. Finally they turned their attention to Kay Parker. Kay had been Matron of Yass Hospital before joining the Army Service and held the most Senior rank among the Army girls. She was six feet tall, exceptionally tall for a girl, and a source of intrigue to these short Japanese men. They walked around her, the dialogue continued, jabbering and grunting while looking her up and down. One Jap brought a stool and placed it at Kay's feet, jumped up on it and looked earnestly into her face. Apparently mollified he hopped down and the pair left without any further ado. Outside they urinated against the wall, "marking their territory like a dog" was the way Whytie put it.[3]

The Army girls told us too of the arrival of the Japs shortly after the landing. They were all lined up expecting to be shot, they said, because the Japs would not acknowledge them as nurses. Some of their able patients were taken away by the Japs and not seen again and at that time it was better not to speculate on what might or might not have been their fate.

After the surrender of Rabaul, the Army doctors of the Field Ambulance Unit gathered the ambulances, medical supplies and orderlies and left, to seek out the men who had taken refuge in the bush. In the ensuing weeks these doctors and orderlies gave valuable assistance to the fleeing troops, and yet later at inland Mission stations. There was increasing deterioration among the men in the harsh conditions, and weakness from lack of food followed constant bouts of fever. Many suffered painful wounds yet, while these could be treated, they endeavoured to persevere in a bid for freedom. The Army nurses were left, safeguarded on Mission premises, where there were Mission and Administration doctors in attendance, yet the nurses felt abandoned by this action on the part of their doctors. Chaplain May of the 2/22nd remained with the nurses but the Japs soon moved him to the camp in Rabaul; two orderlies, who had also remained with them, were taken away by the Japs. They, like the patients, were never seen again.[4]

Our days now became filled with the plodding of army boots on gravel paths and the unnecessary bellow of *Tenko*, accompanied by grunts and guffaws in an effort to make an impact - presumably to back up their lack of stature. Added to the clamour was the gleam of fixed bayonets swinging dangerously about. The commotion caused by this dreaded announcement of their arrival was out of all proportion to the size of the rickety, gaitered legs of the individuals producing it. In these islands monkeys did not exist and the natives had seen them only in pictures, however, by natural instinct, they described the Japanese soldiers as *all a same man long dewai* (like monkeys in the trees). On coming face to face with the Japs looking like clones in Army uniform, their extraordinary physical smallness was a shock to us all.

We found the Japs highly suspicious and easily provoked. On one occasion, when a hapless old native in the ward was carefully hoarding a quantity of strong-smelling stick tobacco under his pillow, a Jap soldier leapt towards his bed and hit him savagely over the head with the butt of the rifle. The Jap made no attempt to find out what the old native was concealing. Several of our old warriors went to their friend's defence and, to the great surprise of the onlookers, the Jap retreated. This was our first lesson - the beginning of many - in discovering an unpredictable trait in the character of the Japanese. Fortunately, the old native escaped with a minor head wound. Most natives were addicted to smoking and the compressed, short moist sticks of tobacco, imported from America, were a coveted possession. They remained fresh for a long time and in the village a 'smoke' was enjoyed most when shared among friends.

As each day passed the missionaries continued to bring in men, unable to proceed, to our hospital and the Army unit. The Administration unit had three doctors now, with the addition of young Doctor Hay, brought across by the Japanese from one of the out-stations. Doctor Watch made an invaluable contribution, but after a short while he and Doctor Hosking were recalled to the Rabaul camp, where medical assistance was needed with the numbers of ailing increasing as more and more captured escapees were brought there by the Japs. Of great concern to us was the fate of Dorothy Maye on Kavieng, we had not received any news of her, and we knew that New Ireland had fallen on the same day as New Britain.

Our small ward overflowed. The convalescent patients were sent upstairs to join the other men and the nursing staff slept down-stairs now, in the ward with the patients. During the night there never seemed to be much disturbance overhead but, in our department, it was bedlam. The guards scarcely left us alone mockingly trying to kiss us. They do not kiss their own women but had probably seen kissing on some European movie and thought it very funny. Just as we were trying to get a little rest they would sidle up to us in the dark and touch us. When we protested, they would twist our arms or clout us over the head and scurry away as though frightened. Maybe they were! The guards were undeniably frightened of their superiors and we thought, hopefully, that since they retreated so readily from our rebuffs they may have been given orders *not* to molest us.

During the day we could not remain seated for long, every time a guard cast his shadow in our vicinity we were required to spring to our feet and bow. To the Japs bowing did not merely mean bowing our heads, but from a standing upright position, we were to bend forward slowly, and while so doing slide our hands down the front of our legs until we were bent over from the hips - the correct way to be polite or appear to be polite, in our case, to our would-be *Masters*. Without doubt this bow was meant to be most profound and gave an inflated aura of exaltation to these Japanese guards of humble parentage. We were becoming increasingly aware that, among the Japs, this habitual bowing of varying manner had a lot to do with degree and rank, and since the rank of the Jap guards was on a low scale they revelled in being the recipients of this sham homage from their prisoners.

Even when we went to the lavatory a guard had to be passed and at times, when the Jap on duty was bored, we'd be given a special lesson in this crazy performance. One day when this occurred I lost my temper and moved off without being dismissed and just ducked the sprightly swing of his arm. Instead of being hauled back and given the thrashing I thought inevitable he just laughed. It took us some time to learn that the Japanese invariably act contrary to what one might expect.

Men kept coming in from the bush every day to seek shelter at the Mission. Running the entire length of this long, narrow island is a very rugged mountain range, a challenge at the best of times to cross. The soldiers had no knowledge of the terrain and groups had many times gone back on their tracks eluding ever increasing Japanese patrols and battling the constant rain of this wet season, with swollen rivers worsening their plight. Many found it impossible to endure.

The refugees had news given them by natives of the fortunate ones who had been picked up by flying-boat or island schooner on the south coast. Some groups had reached comparative safety in the bush after managing to get through the jungle, across the swift flowing rivers and finally, the mountains. Mary was sure that Tom was out there somewhere and she knew he too, would be anxious for news of her. The natives also gave grim news of mass executions in the villages by the Japs for no real reason, other than suspicion. There was a command issued to the natives, they said, to show delight in the Japanese by saluting all Jap soldiers who had come to give protection and salvation to them on their island.

There was another decree, issued to the Australians, immediately after the landing: "Surrender at once and you will be treated as war prisoners, resist and you will be killed one and all". Many weeks later, we were appalled to learn of an atrocious and tragically cruel incident, which happened on the south coast of New Britain on the 4th February. On that day over one hundred and fifty soldiers and civilians who had given no resistance to capture were brutally massacred by the Japanese at Tol Tol Plantation. In four separate executions the escapees, with hands tied behind their backs, were either bayoneted or shot. It was by some miracle that a handful of wounded soldiers escaped and could give account of this gruesome story, and let it be known to all that the Japanese must never be underestimated.[5] The massacre at Tol was kept secret at that time for fear of recrimination, and it was never revealed to Mary Goss.

Around the beginning of February we were fortunate to make the acquaintance of a 3rd Class Japanese private who appeared on guard duty one day and announced he was a Christian, not a highly regarded religion in Japan. He intimated that he was prepared to be helpful to us - he also spoke understandable English. This happy little man had a swaggering cavalier air about him and the men in the camp referred to him as the Laughing Brigand. Tentatively we told him about his colleagues' conduct towards us and, to our surprise, he said he would restrain them when he was on duty.

'Tonight you sleep,' he said, drawing himself up to his full four feet eleven inches that first night he appeared on guard duty. And sleep we did, that night and whenever he was on duty.

At last the men managed to persuade the Japs to let us move our sleeping quarters upstairs where we hoped to have more peace. This arrangement worked much better in spite of the overcrowding which really did make the upstairs floor look like a refugee camp. During sleeping hours bodies protruded from under benches, on top and under tables and even on the stairs. We slept on canvas stretchers on the verandah. Two Australian priests, Father McCullagh and Brother Brennan, had a cosy niche at the top of the stairs, with their heads resting on their swags inside a cupboard. The pair were brought in from one of the Mission's outposts and were kept separate from the other missionaries because they were Australian. They were interned with us as prisoners of war.

With so many people and limited space some organisation was necessary so a committee was formed and duties allocated. One of the happier decisions was the selection of Max Abbott, the Seventh Day Adventist Superintendent, to be our liaison officer. He was a cheerful, tactful man who knew a little Japanese and smoothed the way on several occasions when things looked like getting nasty. He slept on boards, with a few blankets as a mattress, under a window on our verandah dormitory and assured us that boards were a healthy substitute as a bed foundation. When the Japanese were not too much in evidence Max entertained us with amusing stories of his life as a missionary and *other tales* as he called them; these, we suspected, he improvised as he went along. Others soon entered into the spirit of entertainment and contributed their pieces, singing ditties and songs or telling simple Australian yarns.

A week of exceptionally hot, humid weather made conditions in the ward more difficult and an outbreak of dysentery added to our troubles. Worst of all at this time, however, was the shortage of food. A new sanitary bin, for cooking, was supplied by the Mission and an open fireplace set up outside. Food was sent over by the Mission Sisters, but this state of affairs could not go on indefinitely as no supplies were coming in. The Japanese authorities ordered the Mission to send us only the bare necessities which did not include bread. Our diet contained a lot of scraped coconut, which was rich and delicious, but did nothing to help the dysentery sufferers.

Our patients confined to bed were decreasing, but outpatients were increasing as stray natives, and even Japanese, straggled in for treatment of mostly minor ailments. There was no waterborne sewerage at Vunapope either and the men had a rota system for lavatory attendants or, as the Japanese referred to them, *Benjo* men - a most unsavoury occupation by any name!

Baffling problems arose among the Japs guarding us when the oncoming guard could not balance his numbers with the numbers of his predecessor. Counting, we had found from the beginning, was not one of the guards' strong points and there was chaos when changes in our number got too much for them. Almost every day someone had to be exchanged to the ward below, due to malaria or some other emergency, and the resultant, simple additions and subtractions threw the guards into a frenzy. They would move furiously around brandishing ever-ready bayonets and scream *Tenko* at the most unnecessary times of day or night.

Many of our men had grasped a smattering of Japanese by now and some of the more diplomatic among them managed to convince the almost demented Japs that no one had escaped the clutches of the diligent soldiers of *Dai Nippon*. Men had been transferred to the hospital ward, to prevent the terrible disease, from which they were suffering, from spreading, and thereby not endangering the life of everyone, including the Japanese themselves. This simple explanation usually soothed them until new guards arrived and the performance was likely to start all over again to a greater or lessor degree depending on their mathematical talents.

One of our members however did manage to escape, or more correctly, disappear. He was Irish and of course called Paddy; he protested many times that as he was Irish he was neutral and the Japs had no jurisdiction over him. One morning he just walked out and we never saw him again. When *Tenko* came around, in spite of all the fuss surrounding it, the Japs did not even miss him.

The Jap guards never tired of annoying their unresponsive prisoners and harassing the patients, which was fraught with danger when it involved the natives whose reactions could never be predicted. One day when I was on duty a young guard tried to annoy me by catching geckos and putting them in my hair and down the neck of my uniform. An old native who had been shot in the buttocks got awkwardly to his feet and shook his fist at the Jap.

'You no talk all a same long Sister, you no good liklik man long Japan. You shoot im arse long me, liklik taim now balus long America e kom, bombom. You die finish!' To demonstrate how the guard would come to an end the old man threw himself on the bed and gave a realistic display of a victim in his death throes.

The Jap was not angered, but looked afraid at what he took to be an exhibition of insanity, and hurriedly left the ward. We had noted this response before and it did not take us long to realise that the Japanese have not only a fear of mental illness, but an innate fear of the signs of this affliction! Another phobia with them which we did nothing to dispel was that of infectious diseases. When it suited us, we hung a yellow sheet (which they knew meant quarantine) in places where we kept our medical stocks and other things in short supply.

Slapping us across the face was a triumph the guards really enjoyed and we had come to anticipate the indignity as something we were to encounter daily. The bigger and taller among us raised the ire of the Japs more readily, yet without provocation on our part. At first, these face slapping episodes aroused almost uncontrollable fury, not only of the recipients but the onlookers as well. Before too long, however, the sight of a monkey-like figure dancing around like a wrestler getting into position for attack, and often bringing a stool to get nearer his objective, brought on fits of not always silent laughter. We showed no fear and our would-be masters were completely disconcerted. When things were going very badly, we would break into song which annoyed the Japs, and baffled them also.

Face slapping was not dealt out to prisoners alone. An Officer would walk up to one of his men and, for reasons not apparent to us, swipe him across the face. Not the slightest sign of resentment was shown on the face of the Japanese subordinate - perhaps he didn't dare! A truly unpredictable people.

The Japanese guards were a mixed bunch. Many, mostly very young peasants, were curiously childish and quite subdued, while others were aggressive and vicious. As the days passed we were finding it necessary, depending on the mentality of the guards on duty, to keep ourselves segregated from the men. To be seen associating with them would invite obscene gestures, accompanied by suggestive remarks, the latter made worse by broken and crude English.

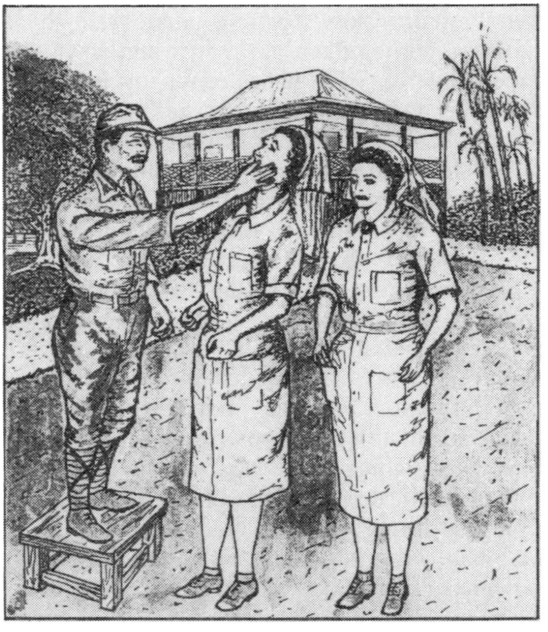

Face slapping - something the guards really enjoyed

Sometime earlier we had received news that, following the occupation of the island, the Japanese Commander had called to see the Bishop of Rabaul at his residence in Vunapope. This visit gave birth to the conjecture that the Japanese High Command had come to some arrangement with the Bishop, regarding the actions of Jap soldiers. Bishop Scharmach was born in Poland but was, in fact, German, and his German leanings gave significant credibility to our theory. The Bishop came to the Sacred Heart Mission in New Guinea from Germany in 1925 and was appointed Bishop of the Diocese in 1939, which, at that time, might have been a clever diplomatic appointment considering the Mission's German ties.

The Sacred Heart Mission was grateful to the Australian authorities for not interning German missionaries at the onset of war with Germany. A good number of the missionaries, who were from different parts of Europe, were aliens, but loyal solely to their cause as missionaries and therefore not the enemy, although there were a few who had gone to the Diocese in Sydney to 'sit-out' the war years. As far as anyone in the camp knew, no specific orders were issued to the Japanese troops, yet, to date, they had not been unduly aggressive towards us. Agreement was unequivocal among our community, that we would do nothing, by word or deed, to upset the *status quo* even though we deemed our situation to be always potentially explosive.[6]

The Japs were removing our patients to the camp in Rabaul as soon as they were showing signs of recovery; a practice abhorrent to us but which we were powerless to do anything about. The intervals between the times when they were taken away and the admission of others brought in by the missionaries were days of enforced idleness. We were all hungry and bored and a great deal of restraint was sometimes necessary to avoid petty bickering, which I thought must have been a natural irritation with so few confined together in uneasiness. Now, too, the guards had more time on their hands as they were not involved with so much mathematical juggling during *Tenko*. A pattern was set for us of work, frustration, boredom and hunger, and frequent harassment by the Japanese.

A particularly diminutive Japanese appeared on the scene one day and was introduced as the *Interpreter*, Sugai San.

'I have been sent by my superiors to report on conditions in this camp and you must all obey,' These opening words must have been a rehearsed 'piece' for would-be interpreters as it was heard (with slight variations) untold times in the years ahead.

After listening to complaints about lack of food and the adverse behaviour of the guards, he informed us, rather pompously, that, in war, soldiers cannot be controlled. Without further ado he left and we wondered what purpose his visit served other than his own.

During our idle hours we had a great need for reading matter and much searching in cupboards brought forth *Pat's Third Term*, read by many schoolgirls. Another, a little more interesting, described the privations of Christopher Columbus and his starving marines on a West Indian island, but the third one unearthed raised a laugh. It was the story of a young couple in love caught up in similar circumstances to our own, but set in Europe during the First World War. The hero consoled the heroine with the promise of taking her to a safe place, like New Guinea, should there ever be another war. He was confident she would not come to any harm in a place like that.

'Were expectations so much different, after all?' we asked ourselves; this was *another war* and New Guinea was far from a *place like that*.

We received our first real disappointment when the Laughing Brigand appeared one day wearing a camouflaged uniform, but not his usual boisterous, good-natured manner.

'Have you come to guard us today?' We asked.

'No, no guard any more. I say goodbye, I go bush catch Scanlan.'

We never saw this helpful character again and, curiously, around this time the Australian Commander surrendered and was taken to a camp in Rabaul to be interrogated.

The worst day so far in our disoriented lives followed the Brigand's departure. It began early one morning when two guards ordered all our able-bodied men to gather their belongings and line up. After a cursory count of heads our companions were marched away without explanation. During the endless time that followed scarcely anyone spoke. The older men, who were left behind, tried to reassure us that perhaps they were being moved to another camp or simply taken on a work-party - something that had not happened before - but, if so, why with all their belongings?

Around midday one of the guards returned. We jumped to our feet as he came into the ward, bowed intuitively as one and waited with uneasy caution as he stood and looked about him. Eventually he grunted and beckoned us outside.

'Bring food!' he said, pointing his rifle at the table.

We collected all the food we could scrounge and a bucket of water and followed him across the grounds of the Mission. Suddenly we came across a sight prompting us to stop, tense with fear, but somehow we kept going not wanting to give vent to our emotions in front of the Jap. Lined up behind the coconut palms, in the hot steaming sun, stood the men who had left us this morning. Their faces were haggard and grey and they hardly seemed to be aware of our presence. At their feet was a newly dug trench. Not a word was spoken by either side as the guards grunted and indicated that their captives could eat. Knowing by now how irrational the Japs could behave, we were by no means reassured by this gesture, nor the order for us to leave.

Back in our quarters the shock had set in and we dared not put into words what we were thinking - 'the Japs have made the men dig their own graves and were going to shoot them'. This method of execution, we had come to know, was practiced by the Japanese and was not at all the exception. We were terrified and entered into a long period of intense silence.

Later when the interruption came, strange as it seemed, it brought forth involuntary exclamations of sheer relief. It was not the gunfire of an execution squad, but the raucous sound of drunken Japanese soldiers!

These off duty Japs had apparently found a liquor supply and were now roaming about so drunk that most of them could not remain on their feet. They followed us around swigging from bottles, the tops of which they had broken off. They certainly had our attention as any minute we expected them to fall on the knifelike glass and all the while our thoughts were concentrated on what action we might take if this were to happen.

'Japanese soldiers take Hong Kong, Guam, New Guinea, now take Australia.'

'You like Japanese soldiers? Soon you go home,' suggested one, while offering a drink from his bottle. Thankfully, their interest in us waned and they began chanting marching songs.

After a while we could hear them stumbling about in other rooms overturning beds and slamming cupboard doors in a frantic search for more liquor. We decided some action on our part was urgently needed. Mary and Grace kept watch while the rest of us made what we hoped was an unobtrusive exit to a nearby room where supplies of liquor were kept for emergency. There seemed no way to stop the Japs from finding this stock and although this was an emergency of a different kind we deemed that what we were about to do was absolutely necessary. However, as we emptied bottles of the best Scotch into a bucket of disinfectant, we were not without misgivings over this sacrilege, especially when we contemplated what the reactions of the men would be. On the way to the outside lavatory two drunks stopped us and pointed to the bucket.

'Byoki (sick)!' I said and disappeared quickly behind the yellow cloth hanging over the entrance. Drunk as they were these two recognised the quarantine sign and kept out.

Over an hour passed. The Japs became tired of looking for booze and further amusements and most of them lurched away - the rest, too drunk to get to their feet, fell asleep where they were.

There was still no sign of the men. Were we to see them

again? One important thing we learned that day was how truly vulnerable we were at the hands of the Japanese. A revelation became only too apparent to me, that however temporary the present might seem to be, the future I had hoped to share with Noel, uncertain though it was, might possibly never be.

We had just finished getting supper for our patients and making them comfortable for the night when three figures appeared striding down the path, an Army officer, a private and a Jap guard. The officer was a dentist living at the Army hospital and they were in need of a doctor. Four natives had just been brought into the hospital urgently requiring medical attention. They had received bad chest and abdominal wounds when Japanese soldiers fired on them as they were innocently fishing off shore. The Jap guard walked over to look at his drunken compatriots and we gave out the bad news that our doctors were taken with the men this morning; we proceeded to give these two men the story of this day of anguish. It was a relief to have someone to talk to and we hoped they could stay for a while, but the Jap guard was 'on duty' and hustled them off.

'What next?' We asked ourselves as we set to work to rid the place of broken glass and tidy up the widespread mess created by the intoxicated Japs. We addressed these chores with a detached air, our thoughts were too occupied with the events of the day. Quite unexpectedly the crunching sound of footsteps along the coral path made us drop everything and listen. Tall forms appeared from around the corner; our men had come back. The guard left them at the door and excited talking started. To our relief all of them had returned, but they were clearly showing the strain of their experience and it was with some remorse that we confessed why we could not offer them that drink, which we knew they would so dearly love. Natural disappointment followed our confession, and when this abated one or two gallantly said we had done the right thing and asked us to give them an account of the escapades of the drunken Japs.

The men could offer no explanation for their ordeal at the mercy of the Japs and they did not know why those threatening trenches were needed. Just after we left them this afternoon, they went on to tell us, they were taken to a deserted native gaol. The guard shoved them inside where there was only standing room and locked the door. Here, amongst overflowing sanitary buckets and general filth was Paddy seemingly unharmed and strangely cheerful. He told them that after leaving the Mission three days earlier he had been accosted on his way to Rabaul by a party of prowling Japs, who fired a shot over his head and wrenched a ring from his finger.

'They wouldn't listen to me when I told them I was neutral and they clapped me in this hell of a calaboose.'

'However,' Paddy went on, 'before the Japs left they handed me a tin of bully beef and one of them even opened it for me with his bayonet. They brought me a bucket of water and locked me in. And I'd not set eyes on anyone at all until you coves came along. But!' he added, 'I will tell you something they didn't find out. Just before they caught me I gave a native two bob for a bottle of whisky, not Irish mind you, but whisky just the same, which I rolled up in my blanket. I'd like to shout you blokes but there's not much left now,' he said sadly.

Paddy did not return with the men. Whether the decision was his or the Japs no one knew.

'Good luck to him anyway,' someone murmured, 'he gave us a laugh on this bloody awful day.'

The guards refused to let our doctors go to the Army hospital to see the wounded natives, and we only hoped the Mission doctor had been located.

'Not a good way to win these people over to their cause,' Noel said with scepticism.

'Especially as they profess to be offering protection for them from their white oppressors!' I added.

On the 15th of February the greatest prize of all fell into the hands of the Japanese - impregnable Singapore. Words could not express the paralysed feeling within us on receiving this unbelievable news from one of the missionaries; hopes were instantly vanquished. All Australians were of the opinion that Singapore was a secure island fortress likened to the Rock of Gibraltar, that invincible British fortress in the Mediterranean whose name is synonymous with impregnability and already proving itself in this war as it has done for centuries past. Would there ever be an end to the advance of the Japanese? And how safe now was Port Moresby?

Towards evening pandemonium broke loose. To celebrate the greatest victory since the untimely attack on Pearl Harbor the Japs played the conquering heroes. Drunken Japs made the night hideous with screams and cheers accompanying Japanese marching songs, but there was one consolation, they kept away from the Mission. And us!

It did not take much now, under all this uncertainty, to cause apprehension over any deviation in the daily routine. Another morning, just as we were finishing our meagre breakfast of tea and porridge, a vehicle pulled up near the building and a rather spruce looking Japanese officer walked up to Pastor Abbott and ordered us all to line up. He dismissed the women and older men and beckoned the remainder to follow him. With quiet resignation the men climbed aboard the truck and as they waved to us our thoughts were of a similar day not so long ago and we were stricken again with anxiety.

Just as the sun was setting on this seemingly endless day of worry the truck pulled up outside. To our amazement a group of happy looking men carrying swags over their shoulders tumbled out.

'Look what we've brought you!'

They proceeded to unroll the curtains they had used as swags and after all our distress this day turned out to be fruitful. The officer had taken them on a work-party to clean out the abandoned houses in and around Rabaul. Many houses, by happy chance, had not been fully stripped of all their former owners' goods and the Japanese officer had been quite a good sport and allowed the men to keep some articles from the pilfering. This welcome loot comprised tins of food, cereals, crockery and utensils, native tobacco and even a mincer and, wonder of wonders, packs of cards. The cards turned out to be a great boon and were so much in demand that it wasn't long before they were in need of a facelift.

A former dapper man about town, now wearing a *laplap*, set up the kitchen mincer. He was joined by our young doctor clad in a pair of cast-off shorts - not dressed in his usual pristine style either. Our present state brought to light some ill-assorted modes of dress and left no room for inhibitions. These two were sweating profusely while trying to turn *native twist* into *fine cut* and, being urged on with encouraging advice from the local wits, they made us all forget our troubles, temporarily. After it had been treated that tobacco was appreciated by the desperate smokers.

Next morning Joyce, Lik, Grace and I were trying to bring some order into the upstairs dormitory when we noticed several derelict cars parked below. The Japanese were tinkering with the vehicles and we joined a few of our men who were standing around watching.

When we came closer it was apparent that the men looked amused and we soon saw why. The Japs were running around like circus clowns alternately cranking and peering short-sightedly into the engines. Adding to the comedy large stones had been placed near the cars to give the Japs more height in order to take a closer look. As spectators we were completely ignored. In these early days of captivity we had not yet come to know that all Japanese have a one track mind. Today it was on cars.

'How these galahs ever get their planes into the air beats me.'

This was just one of the many remarks we heard before we discreetly returned to our quarters.

A few days later the cars had disappeared and horses took their place under the trees and it was another day of entertainment for the onlookers. Though some missionaries and plantation owners rode horses these animals were virtually unknown in the islands, and the fact that they had come complete with bales of hay suggested that they must have been brought in by sea. The Australians nearly went into hysterics when the bow-legged little soldiers lined the horses up against a wall and jumped, like stunt riders, on to their backs. Our fertile minds switched to the movies, but found it somewhat hard to envisage scenes of *Japanese* heroes tying their cloth-wrapped bundles to saddles and cantering off into the distance.

Apart from these lighter interludes many in the camp did keep an interested eye on the movements of the enemy. There was wide speculation as to whether these horsemen were going into the bush to locate the remnants of our defeated Army or, whether the horses were to be used by the Japs to seek an access route over the Owen Stanley mountains of the mainland, which would need to be crossed if Port Moresby could not be taken by sea. Port Moresby was apparently the only obstacle in the way of a Japanese advance on Australia. How were they faring in Australia?

Soon after the fall of Singapore we had a strange invasion at Vunapope which caused a considerable stir among us all. One morning after breakfast we looked out from the upstairs verandah to see a moving mass of colour spreading from the lawn below us to the front of the cathedral. There were hundreds of tiny women in bright *kimonos* flitting about like swarms of butterflies and everyone who could move was fixed on the sight.

'Where have they come from?'

'They came from Japan by ship.'

'No! The Americans dropped them in by parachute to keep the Japs busy while they, the Yanks that is, get on with their invasion plans.'

Opinions varied and ranged from the obvious to the ridiculous. When the excitement died down the conclusion most vital about the advent of the *Girls* was that, in keeping their countrymen entertained, their presence will surely be beneficial to us.

Opposite our residence was a three-storey building where the Brothers of the Mission lived and it was painfully clear that they were moving out. Missionaries from the building were carrying cases and baggage; we spotted Father Barrow, whom we'd met at Christmas, reduced to an undignified role among the porters. While the *Girls* waited demurely on the lawn, the Japs looked on from a distance.

As the last of the Brothers left their home, the visitors on the lawn gathered up their handkerchief bundles and hurried inside. We felt a deep sympathy for the missionaries over this humiliation, yet, at the same time gained comfort from the realisation that, with so many of their own women on the premises, the Japanese would no longer pay undue attention towards us. We at least fervently hoped!

On the afternoon of the Day of the Girls, as we came to call this event, there was more activity. The horses that were stabled in, of all places, the cathedral were led out, followed by large bundles of hay, after which a cleaning squad moved in. When all was in readiness a solemn procession was formed headed by the very top brass, with their long swords dangling, followed by the Navy and Army and their respective Air Forces and the *Girls* bringing up the rear. We were informed that this was a service (Shinto or Buddhist or a combination of the two, no one quite knew) for the brave Japanese soldiers killed during the taking of Rabaul.[7]

The cathedral had already been desecrated when it was used as a stable and now it was being further defiled by what could only be regarded, by our Christian missionaries, as a pagan ceremony. It did seem bizarre that the Japs saw fit to hold such a service in a Christian cathedral and we wondered what the thoughts of the missionaries might be. Since the occupation began, use of the cathedral was forbidden and all religious work of the Mission was suppressed by the Japanese. The Japanese had no regard for Christian religion and demanded of the missionaries and their native catechists throughout New Britain that Christianity must be wiped out in the Pacific.[8]

A few days later, Mr McEwan, a messenger from the Rabaul camp, arrived at the Mission under Japanese escort. Mr McEwan was the grocery manager of Rabaul's Burns Philp store and a Sergeant in the New Guinea Volunteer Rifles. He was working with the hospital group at the Rabaul camp and had been sent by Doctor Hosking to obtain as many drugs as possible from our store. So far Doctor Cooper had been able to keep his supply of medicines hidden away from prying Japanese eyes.

While supplies were being sorted out our visitor gave us news of conditions in the Rabaul camp which was by no means encouraging. There was a shortage of food and all other amenities and the guards were ceaselessly troublesome. He told us that groups had been formed among the men to take care of the necessary functions to cater for over a thousand prisoners in the camp, and to keep existing services in Rabaul in working order - for the Japs. Disappointingly he had no news to give Mary of her husband.

The lives of the native people particularly, Mr McEwan said, were made complicated by this war which they could not comprehend. The indigenous people of New Britain suffered from other invaders as well - many thousands of indentured plantation labourers now without employment and unable to return to their homes. The Australian Government insisted that these labourers be recruited from within the Territory and most of them were from the great Sepik River district on the mainland of New Guinea. They were forced by their captors to work for the Japanese secret police, the Kempeitai. The Kempeitai was a military corps, akin to the German Gestapo, with wide and ruthless powers and well trained to use them. The New Guineans were fed only small rations of rice and locked up at night; they were virtually imprisoned. Those who escaped and fled to the bush were not welcomed by the villagers who had already seen their food supplies depleted by roving Japanese and streams of soldiers and civilians fleeing after the capitulation of Rabaul. A penalty of death was imposed on anyone stealing food from the Japs and this execution was carried out mercilessly by decapitation with the sword. The people were in fear of the unpredictable Japanese.

The Chinese did not fare any better either, so many atrocious stories were told following the days of the Japanese landing. Some Chinese eked out a bare existence on deserted plantations while others were forced to run eating houses for their Japanese *liberators*. The Chinese women of course did not escape, the Japanese being far more attracted to these close relatives than to other races. They considered the native women repulsive and unclean but changed their minds as time passed, so we were told.

The day after Mr McEwan's visit Doctor Cooper appeared wearing a grave expression, an open letter in his hand.

'I am afraid I have very bad news - Angela Choy has to go back to her own people in Rabaul.' We had grave fears for Angela.

These were anxious times. With Singapore gone and the Japanese virtually masters of the Pacific conjecture and rumours were rife. The only scraps of news we could rely on came from the men who were brought in by the missionaries. Most of them had been in recent contact with those still free who were illicitly operating wirelesses.

Towards the end of February, Doctor Cooper told us that there had been rumours we were all to be taken to Rabaul and, therefore, it would be wise to distribute among ourselves the remaining medical supplies. We would be more likely to get away with essential drugs and first-aid equipment if stored in individual kit-bags, he said. Doctor Cooper was a diabetic and was dependant on insulin daily and we were constantly worried about his welfare as stocks of this essential drug diminished. Joyce and I believed that he should have been evacuated in December, though we knew how dedicated he was to his profession and would never have considered leaving his post.

Much in evidence these days was a nasty little Japanese doctor called Chikami - and referred to by our men as Sunshine Sam. Just how diabolical and cold-blooded he was we were to learn. He was responsible for an atrocity, in face of all others, hard to believe. Captain Gray of Engineer Services had been captured by the Japs soon after the fall of Rabaul. He refused to give information about the Australian Army and was tied to a tree near the Bishop's residence, a residence which was now occupied by the Japanese Army officer in charge of the Japs at Vunapope, Lieutenant Colonel Kuata. After brutal interrogation Captain Gray was repeatedly beaten, but his courage was entwined in the fibres of his heart and his torturers could gain no information from him. He was taken to a nearby coconut plantation where missionaries were forced to witness his macabre execution. Doctor Chikami cut out this brave man's heart while he was still alive "in order to study his reactions".[9]

Since the advent of the *Girls*, now living in the former residence of the Brothers, Doctor Chikami was zealously engrossed in *treating* them. Daily he could be seen with instruments in his hands - no black bag for him - crossing the lawns to their quarters. Having not much else to do we speculated on the problems those poor girls might have and how ghastly their collective fate. We wondered how so many had come to be mixed up in this war. We did not know, at that time, that most of them were taken by force into their degrading occupation and that the majority of them were not of Japanese origin.[10]

Our medical supplies would certainly be lost to us if the infamous Japanese Doctor Chikami knew of their existence. The distribution of drugs as suggested by Doctor Cooper proved to be a wise decision.

4

VUNAPOPE - CONVENT

The rainy season was beginning to show signs of coming to an end and on this crisp morning of 25th February the light cool breeze, that always came in from the sea, was generously distributing the tropical aroma throughout the buildings.

'A fine morning for turning out the ward and getting some laundry done,' Mary said as she and Joyce energetically stripped beds and overturned mattresses.

Although the sick and injured were still being brought here by the missionaries the numbers in the ward had decreased drastically. Earnest pleas from Doctor Cooper to keep the patients with us were disregarded. We knew they could be much better cared for at Vunapope than in the camp at Rabaul but the Japanese demanded they be moved, often before they were recovered.

Our guard was mostly inconspicuous this morning and in the generally relaxed atmosphere the inmates, as some of the men referred to themselves, were involved in making our living quarters more habitable. One month had passed since our capture and so much had happened in those weeks it was hard to believe that only four had gone by.

Taking advantage of the absence of the guards, a few of our particular friends were giving us a hand with our ward work. Whistling and snatches of song came from the ablution block where other workers were trying to take their minds off the unsavoury chores in that area. All this make believe atmosphere ended when a Japanese officer arrived. He went directly to Doctor Cooper and, as he talked, waved his hands in our direction. When Doctor Cooper came towards us the cheerful work group plunged into deadly silence - something ominous was about to happen.

'You girls are to go with this officer, but don't worry, I think he is taking you to the Convent. Take all the medical supplies you can manage and ...' he broke off as the officer shrieked *hayaku*. The use of Japanese on this occasion obviously to create an aura of fear.

'Good luck.' These were the last words we heard as the officer herded us outside.

With the characteristic callous attitude of our captors we were granted no opportunity to thank our men for their kindness and protection, given so freely before and after we were captured last month. We were consoled only in the realisation that they would have known our gratitude without the expression of words. There was understandable sadness in parting and no one spoke as the six of us were marched across crunching coral paths and velvet smooth lawns to the open doors of the Convent.

'We're so pleased to see you. We have been asking the Japanese from the beginning to let you girls join us here.'

This warm greeting from the nuns gladdened our hearts and helped me overcome anguished feelings following the abrupt parting from Noel. The kindness of these missionary sisters was overwhelming and we were almost speechless when seated at a table, covered with a starched white tablecloth, laden with bread, dripping and jam, and the greatest treat of all - tea with milk! After we had feasted the nuns told us that they still had a fairly well stocked store and began to relate how this came about. The Irish nuns took up the tale.

With the imminent landing of the Japs the manager of the Kokopo Burns Philp store had handed the missionary sisters the key and given them permission to take anything from the store they might need. The Irish nuns offered to do the shopping, claiming that they were neutral and the Japanese would not touch them should they make an appearance. With native helpers a lorry was hurriedly loaded with everything it was possible to carry and just as the nuns were returning to the Mission the Japanese swarmed ashore at Kokopo. At that stage the Japs had more to concern themselves with than to pursue a lorry load of nuns and natives, and so the shopping party was allowed to proceed unmolested. Nevertheless, the Irish nuns had their own version of the episode and firmly believed they were spared only because the Japanese knew they were neutral!

We couldn't help telling these Irish ladies about our man Paddy, who believed as well that he was neutral and ended up in a native gaol among the sanitary pails. Reluctantly, we had to admit that we were never able to find out what eventually became of him. Where in the Japanese scheme of things did his neutrality belong?

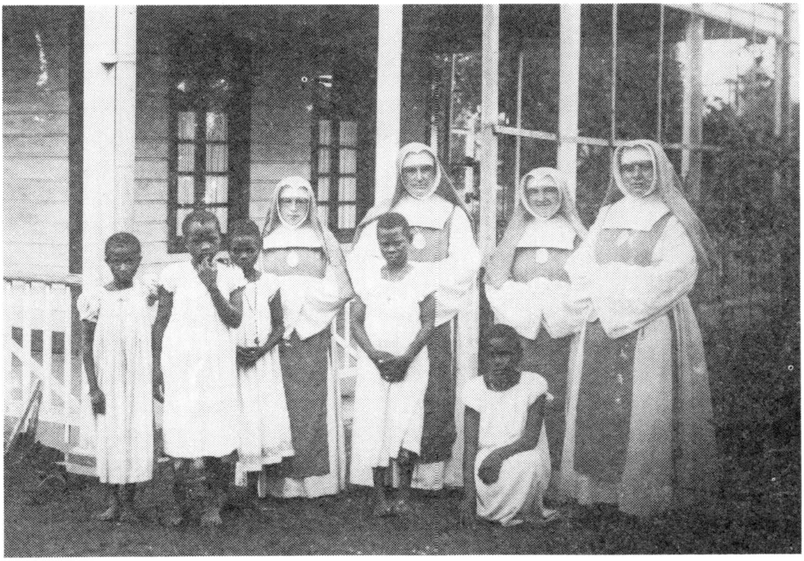

Australian Sisters of Our Lady of the Sacred Heart

This part of the Convent complex housed the Australian, Dutch, French and Irish nuns. Since the invasion the six Army girls had been given shelter here as well as the four Methodist missionary nurses (Mavis Green, Dora Wilson, Jean Christopher and Dorothy Beale) who had elected to stay. They were from the Mission hospital at Malabunga, a few miles along the road from Vunakanau Airport. We were surprised to see Mrs Kathleen Bignell in this group. Mrs Bignell was a plantation owner with a long association in New Britain and the Solomon Islands. She had chosen against evacuation. Her son was somewhere on the island working with a timber company; after searching in vain for him she was captured only a few days ago and brought to Vunapope. There were, apparently, two or three other plantation women who did not leave the island in December when the women were evacuated. To date their fate remains unknown.

After morning tea the six of us, Mrs Bignell and the Methodist nurses were settled in to our new quarters. In the evening Father Barrow paid us a visit. We did not know then what a friendly liaison officer the good Father was to become. He was the former parish priest in Rabaul and was what one might call a typical Irishman, cheerful and stockily built. He had been captured in the general round-up of civilians soon after the landing and, during the process of sorting out different nationalities, he was eventually labelled neutral by the Japs and sent to Vunapope Mission.

'I'm sorry to say I have bad news for you girls - the men you were with have all been taken to the camp in Rabaul and interned with the other civilians and Army personnel. The Japanese are putting them to work on the waterfront.'

This was grave news. Their safety was paramount and while working for the enemy, on such likely targets as the waterfront, they would be exposed to the frequent bombing raids of their Allies; the scales of justice were unethically out of balance. We had lost contact with the men altogether, but we unashamedly confessed relief that we had not been ordered to Rabaul as was previously rumoured. We only hoped that Doctor Cooper was able to remove the remaining stocks of medical supplies in the cupboards of our former quarters, although this seemed unlikely with the acquisitive Doctor Chikami around.

Settling in at Australia House - a suitable name we gave our quarters - we could scarcely believe the peace and comfort that prevailed. Here we had very hygienic surroundings and adequate food; no ever-present guards and no roll-calls. The nuns spared no effort in making life easier for us. They supplied us with mattresses, chairs, crockery and as many essentials as they possibly could, at the expense of their own comfort we felt quite certain. We formed ourselves into groups to cope more easily with domestic matters.

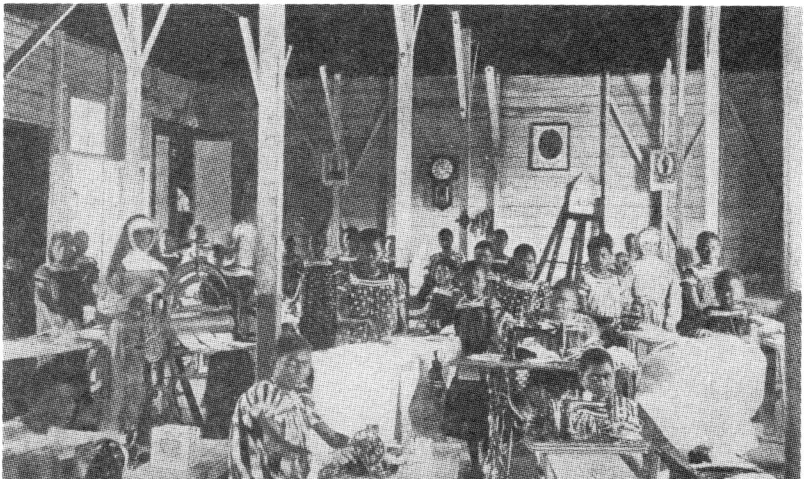

Sewing classes for native girls

Vunapope Mission had been serving the community since 1882. Now, in 1942, there were seventeen different nationalities strengthening the Mission with their expertise, and everything essential for the running of this well organised society was catered for right down to the printing of the Mission newspaper. The missionaries ran native schools and hospitals, manufactured what was necessary for daily living and grew their own vegetables. They were truly self-supporting; for outsiders, like ourselves, now a part of this multi-cultural establishment there was always something new to learn.

Over the years the Mission had helped so many in need. It was at Vunapope that the whole of Rabaul had taken refuge during the 1937 volcanic eruption and again, in this critical time of war, the missionaries were ever ready to give sanctuary without question. The brothers and priests were secretly in wireless communication with scattered Mission posts inland and there, as here, they considered it their duty to seek victims of the invasion who were still holding out and give aid to these sick and, more often now, starving refugees.

An outstanding character at the Mission was Sister Borgia, an Australian nun who was nearly eighty years old. In her long life she had watched the course of change in New Guinea, from German to Australian, experienced a major earthquake and a violent, volcanic eruption and now she was witnessing a mammoth invasion of these islands. The other nuns told us that Sister Borgia was firmly convinced that the Americans would soon be coming to the rescue.

'Thank God the Americans have not come too late!' she passionately exclaimed on beholding the awe-inspiring spectacle of the Japanese invasion fleet making its triumphal entry into the passage that shattering morning of the 23rd January. The other nuns teased the old lady for a considerable time over this outburst, but Sister Borgia proved to be a tough old veteran in those trying times of Japanese domination.[1]

Father Barrow was eager to help us in any way he could. Because of his neutrality he was allowed to travel between the various camps, where he not only observed the functioning of them but gathered as much information as possible from the internees. There were still a few people who secretly possessed radios and Father Barrow, while covertly conducting missionary duties, circulated the latest war news. He carried letters and messages to our friends - we had not lost contact with the men after all. In less than no time the Father became a very busy man, and when he breezily arrived on our territory his thick brogue was the signal for us to drop everything, gather round and listen to his news.

He told us more about the groups formed among prisoners to run the operations of the camp, the hospital group, cooking group and so on, and that from the beginning the Japs had ordered other groups to look after essential installations, namely the *Freezer* plant and power supply. Gordon Thomas the editor of the *Rabaul Times* seemed to be a very worthy liaison officer as well as cook in the *Freezer* group. The troops and civilians were utilised on the wharves to unload the ships which were always coming and going with equipment. It was becoming painfully obvious that Rabaul was an important base for the Japanese Command and would not be given up lightly. The strategic position of New Britain, earned it the title of an unsinkable aircraft carrier.

One day down on the wharf, when the prisoners were unloading cargo, Father Barrow had seen them drop a box of tinned goods and "as quick as a flash", to quote his words, "the box simply disappeared".

'You know, these countrymen of yours have become such experts, I am sure they must have a bit of Ned Kelly in their ancestry.'

The rescue work was still going on deep into the island and the stories were of great suffering and hardship. Pitiful accounts were told by the brothers from the various inland Missions who discovered men, surrounded by dead companions. These survivors asked to be shot rather than surrender to the Japs. They were worn out and in such poor physical condition, yet many of them operated wirelesses in remote plantation houses, hiding in the bush during the day enabling them to broadcast and gather news during the night. They had no quinine to combat malaria and were continually wet from the ever constant rain; only the very fit survived these conditions.

We had a wonderfully happy surprise one day with the appearance at the Mission of Maisie, whose well-being we had not received any news of to date. Dorothy Maye had been in the islands since 1935 and was stationed at Kavieng on the large nearby island of New Ireland. The Japs brought her over to join us at Australia House and Maisie was overjoyed to be with her own kind again. She had experienced some hair-raising and anxious times since the Japanese landing at Kavieng on 23rd January. She was the only white woman at the hospital and after the invasion the Japs transferred her to a house where a Japanese doctor was in residence. She was of course gravely apprehensive but, as the days passed and the doctor kept to his area of the house, she was reassured.

There was one evening, she told us, when a crowd of young Japanese officers arrived and from the awful noise of Japanese music blaring from the wireless it was obvious that the little doctor was entertaining. Just as she was getting used to the din and beginning to doze she felt the mosquito net being pulled out. Jumping up she opened her mouth to scream. It was just as well no sound came forth, Maisie said, for the little doctor just stood beside her bed smiling and handed her a large slice of paw-paw, then, as quietly as he came in, he padded out.

She told us that a Japanese Naval officer spoke to her one day while she was being held captive on New Ireland.

'We have met before - I am very sorry for you Sister Maye,' he said briefly and seemed to bear no animosity.

Many Japanese Naval men visited these islands before war erupted with Japan. Most of us remembered well the sleek Japanese motor ship, the *Takaichiho Maru*. This vessel called at Rabaul quite often; her crew were made welcome in a town they had come to know so well, in a town whose countrymen were part of the prosperous business community before their internment immediately following the bombing of Pearl Harbor. There seemed nothing unusual about the regular visits of the *Takaichiho Maru*; we were not at war with Japan at that time.[2] It was acknowledged sometime later, Father Barrow told us, that on many Japanese ships to visit these waters Japanese Naval Intelligence Officers were engaged among the crew, covertly, as deckhands, thus enabling them to carry out undercover work in Rabaul and other places for the Government of Japan.

The building next to Australia House was a scene of activity every day and often well into the night; it housed the Mission's huge laundry. Not only was the washing from Vunapope undertaken here but a great deal was normally brought in from out-lying Missions as well. There was a section in the laundry with long concrete troughs where the root of the tapioca was turned into Cassava flour. The root was grated into the troughs and soaked in water which was later drained off; the fibre was separated from the starch, dried and sieved several times to produce the final product. This substance was rather sticky, initially, but made delicious bread.

A broad-faced Dutch nun supervised this hive of industry. She became a source of great interest and inspiration to us as the days went by. She told us of her experiences, past and present, in a clear ringing voice and her broken English had a delightful cheerfulness that was better than any tonic for tattered nerves.

'I am not so thick as before,' she informed us one morning after breakfast; her hands rested on an ample waistline and a generous smile spread across her face displaying sparkling white teeth.

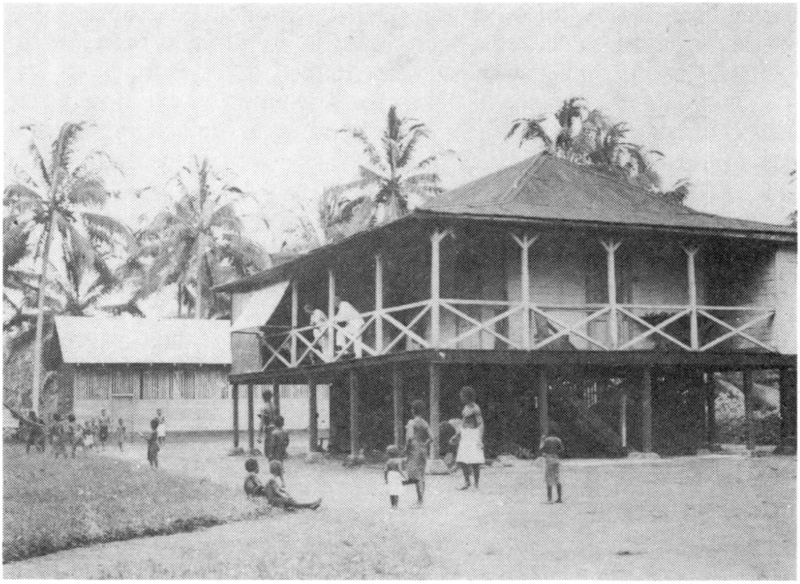

A Mission building

'This morning I had *thirteen* bananas - only little ones *now*. But it is just not the same as bread and butter with cheese; not even your Australian cheese *now*.' She rolled her eyes, shrugged her shoulders and laughed. 'Never mind, not today, perhaps tomorrow.'

'Yes,' we smiled 'not now, tomorrow.' *Tomorrow* holds the key - the key to freedom - and we prayed that the dawning of that day would soon come. We called our Dutch neighbour Sister Matilda since her presence always brought us glad thoughts of home.

'What name is it?' she asked.

'Well, it is a very special Australian ballad and as you are such a happy person we thought Matilda would be a nice name for you.' I said with some uncertainty. Australians have long been inspired by the strains of Waltzing Matilda written to Banjo Paterson's prose and she was delighted. Centred around happenings in the days of the great shearer's strike in Queensland's outback last century, and extraordinarily patriotic, Waltzing Matilda laments the story of an ill-fated swagman camped by a billabong, which, as legend decrees, was in that part of far western Queensland where I grew up.

Matilda sent her native girls over to teach us how to scrape coconut meat from the hard shell. They brought with them a narrow board on the end of which was attached a metal scraper. The demonstrator sat on the flat end of the board on a low stool and vigorously shredded the broken coconut shell over the scraper into a bowl in front of her. A thick creamy milk was obtained by wringing the contents several times through muslin. This very rich, delicious coconut cream could be used for cooking yams, taro and sweet potatoes wrapped in leaves and baked in an earth-oven, and when poured over tropical fruit it created a mouth-watering desert.

Throughout all this activity we were not entirely free of the Japanese presence. There were frequent visits by Jap soldiers who would descend from vehicles and prowl around the buildings especially the laundry and outbuildings. We did our utmost to avoid them though we were not always successful.

'You like Japanese soldier? You come Rabaul sing, drink beer?' were the usual questions asked of us at these times, but they did not become aggressive by our lack of response, much to our relief. One such visit provided us with mild entertainment, however, Sister Matilda did not share the amusement.

On this day, when the Japanese came to visit, our friendly Sister was resting on the upstairs verandah of the Convent. The Japs disappeared into the laundry and emerged, some time later, in the nude and spread themselves on the lawn to bask in the sun. They had seized the opportunity to take a much, no doubt needed bath. Our thoughts on what might be likely to happen next were interrupted by a most un-nunlike bellow from the direction of the Convent - Sister Matilda was quite definitely not amused.

The bathers took no notice of this interruption, neither did the rest of the missionaries and the bathing party eventually dressed and departed without incident.

One day, a few of our former native hospital staff from Rabaul came to visit us. Their treatment at the hands of the Japanese made a sad tale, but their demonstration of some of the antics of our contemporary overlords left us with a smile.

'This man long Japan he sit on graun in haus kuk, he kaikai planti rice thas all, he stink all e wankain (same) pig he die long time before.'

'He walk about all e wankain arse e broke.' This was a crude, though fairly accurate description of a swaggering bandy-legged Japanese soldier. Before they left, these boys seemed anxious to demonstrate how the Japs, not knowing the native language or Pidgin, went about asking for eggs.

'Supossim e like kaikai kiau (egg), e sit down long graun all e wankain mipela kakaruk (fowl).' Waiting a few minutes the actor rose to his feet, flapped his arms about and started making cackling noises. This really got a laugh! When it was time for the boys to leave we could only offer them a few bananas from our diminishing supply.

Our life at Vunapope became almost a pleasure due entirely to the attitude and ingenuity of the nuns. Several of our group had attended Convent schools in Australia and we all agreed that the Sisters at home weren't a bit like these Sisters here. When we got to know them well, I mentioned this to one of the older, more outspoken nuns and she laughed.

'You know in the past nuns from Convents in Australia used to come to Rabaul on holidays, but after a while their visits ceased. When I went down there for my vacation I inquired of the Mother Superior why her group did not visit us any more. She looked a bit embarrassed but was quite a good sport and began to laugh.'

'"Well, we think you are more worldly up there in the tropics and have more advanced ideas than we have. We were of the opinion that our nuns were finding it too difficult after their vacation to settle again into our more strict routine".' quoted the Mother Superior.

We spent many happy hours with the nuns and joined in the plays they organised for entertainment. They arranged commercial courses and language classes for those who were interested, and many a game of deck-tennis was played. To add to their difficulties the Japanese had taken over many of the seventy-eight buildings comprising the Mission, yet the Bishop, priests and nuns decided from the beginning that they would keep their minds occupied in an endeavour to hold morale at a high level in their ever-increasing community. We were naturally of differing religious beliefs among the members of our group, yet we were welcomed equally as were the nurses from the Methodist Mission. These nuns were definitely good sports! Any attempt on our part to express gratitude was airily dismissed with the much used Pidgin expression in these islands.

'It is something nothing.'

On the 26th March, giant planes appeared in the sky over Rabaul and caused a great deal of frenzied activity among the Japs. We had never seen anything like them before; previous raids were with Catalinas. From the excitement created among the Japs these planes were quite definitely something new to them as well. They were the magnificent American Flying Fortresses and this was the greatest air raid on Rabaul since the invasion. It was a wonderful boost to our morale, although it cast grave shadows of anxiety about the safety of our men in the camps.

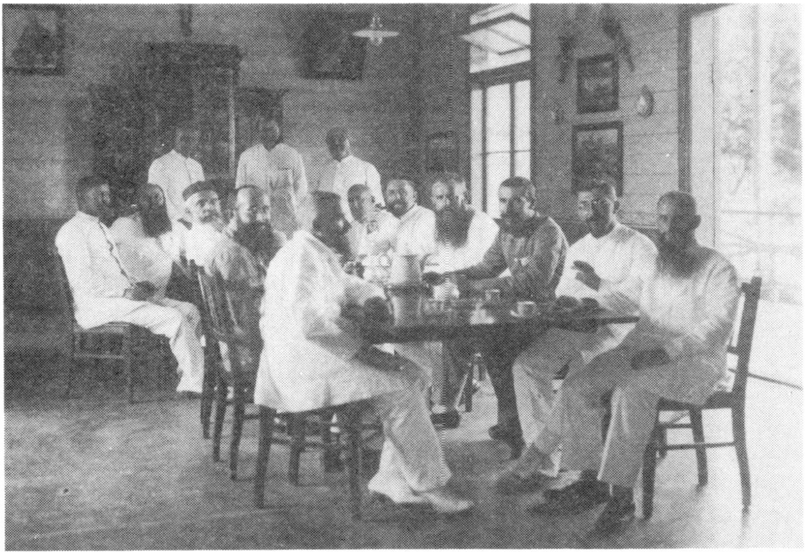

Mission Priests taken before the Second World War
Bishop Scharmach (as a priest), second from right

When Father Barrow arrived next day we knew from his usual breezy manner that all was well. He told us that the raid had done considerable damage to strategic defences, but there had been no damage in the camps in Rabaul, although someone received a near miss when a handle was blown off a cooking pot! We suspected that this was a portrayal of Father Barrow's Irish wit designed to relieve our tension.

More outstanding bombers of the American squadrons, B-26 Marauders, came over in daylight hours. In the middle of April an important Japanese supply ship tied-up at the wharf received a direct hit, when bombed by a low-flying Marauder. Father Barrow's report told us later that the earth-shattering explosion, and consequent fire, was caused by aviation fuel about to be unloaded from the ship. The disastrous fire engulfed the wharf area and raged all day; from Vunapope it had looked to be out of control, threatening Rabaul. There was a further massive explosion after sunset when ammunition loaded in the stern blew up; the ship sank leaving the bow visible above the waterline. Crated aircraft and drums of oil stored around the wharf were destroyed by the fire. On hearing of all the damage we gave three cheers to the Americans.

Raids were coming frequently now, either in the morning or at night and the Japanese were intensifying their reign over New Britain. All nursing duties at Vunapope ceased in April and the hospital in the Mission grounds was closed. Anyone needing medical attention, who was found in the interior, was taken to Rabaul where conditions were primitive to say the least and food in short supply, and where there was always the threat of becoming a casualty from Allied bombing.

Of late, there was a great deal of feverish activity in the harbour. Aircraft carriers, submarines, oil tankers and transports were ceaselessly moving in and out; supplies were unloaded and yet more troops; planes seemed to be on manoeuvres above. One ship, which had remained more or less stationary, we called the Watchdog. It was anchored outside the entrance to Blanche Bay and seemed immune to bombardment from Allied aircraft. From viewing points at Australia House, where we gathered when the ack-ack went into action, we could see the tracer bullets trying to focus on the bombers as they zoomed in over the Upper 'drome and harbour. Our aircraft looked to be, actually, hovering over the Watchdog. We waited eagerly until one night, what we had been hoping for happened!

Loud explosions brought us hastily to our lookouts. Sirens shrieked and the sky over Rabaul was lit as if by sunlight. In the clear light we watched enthralled as the Watchdog shuddered, rolled, and like a giant whale, slowly sank into the sea. This was another exciting raid by the Flying Fortresses. Our spirits were lifted to such great heights by the recent raids that we started taking bets on an imminent American landing and just how soon we would be back in Australia!

Towards the beginning of May we noticed ships moving in convoy out of Rabaul. One convoy of heavy cruisers, heading south, guarded a sleek Jap aircraft carrier; on that day alone, before the light failed, we counted about twenty-seven vessels of various types: cruisers, destroyers, minesweepers and transports.

'Japanese take Moresby, then Australia, you go home,' boastingly stated a few Jap guards.

A mood of tension and foreboding crept into the optimistic environment and for the first time since our capture we became doubtful. We began to wonder whether it would be possible, even with the sort of American help we had witnessed first-hand, to hold off an invasion of Australia if Port Moresby were to fall to the Japanese. Impulsive rumours circulated causing anxiety to mount.

On the days following what we now referred to as the Sailing of the Armada reports were heard about natives being forcibly taken aboard some ships of the fleet. The purpose of this kidnapping, according to Father Barrow, was to use them as interpreters when the Japanese captured Port Moresby. This did not say much for the mentality of the Jap officials. It had apparently not occurred to them, or they did not know, that there were hundreds of different tribes in these islands with as many different dialects.[3]

'"They might just as well have gone to Alaska and picked up a few Eskimos" was a remark put forward by one old-timer,' said Father Barrow. The Father had gathered lots of information and interesting tit-bits about incidents with the island people.

Father Barrow told us of young Japanese soldiers escaping while being transferred to waiting ships, possibly the transports bound for the invasion of Port Moresby. Several were caught, beaten and once more put on board. This tale brought back scenes of our first days at Vunapope when we noticed the Japanese soldiers, who looked to be no older than country school boys, raiding the Mission's fruit trees. It also exploded the myth that all Japanese were willing to die for the Son of Heaven! Every Japanese boy was brought up to believe that the greatest honour that could befall him was to die for his Emperor and country, if need be. His courage was to be matched by his honour in the sacredness of his promise and the impossibility of yielding while life lasts! The devout belief of the Japanese in the code of *Bushido* supported the militarist extremists in a plan of total indoctrination.

Several of us from Australia House were outside enjoying the sea breeze in the mid-afternoon of the 11th May. The Japs had been very quiet for days, depressed was how some rumours described them, though no one could really believe anything said about the Japanese - it was impossible to understand them.

'Look at that out there!' One of the missionary nurses was pointing seaward. Excitement spiralled as the specks on the horizon grew larger and multiplied. The small gathering near the beachfront increased and optimism mounted, without much reason, as it frequently did these days since the appearance of the Flying Fortresses.

'They're Yanks - they cleaned up the Jap fleet before it got to Moresby and here they are!'

This premature euphoria was short-lived. The ships that came into focus were a battered and dirty replica of the fleet that had sailed so jauntily out of Rabaul less than a week ago.

Nothing, however, illustrated defeat more poignantly than the pitiful sight of a wounded aircraft carrier, hugging the shore near Kokopo as it very slowly made its way to anchorage, as an animal to its lair. When this pride of the Japanese Navy - or one bearing her resemblance - set forth for an encounter with the Allied Forces her decks were covered with planes, perched like a flock of gulls on the flat top. Today, the pitted superstructure stood out starkly above the now almost deserted decks, from which the birds had flown and never returned.

As the small crowd on the beach at Vunapope watched the stricken Armada approach from the horizon and limp unpretentiously into Blanche Bay, the significance of the strategic defeat of the Japanese in the Battle of the Coral Sea, by the Americans and Australians, was known only to a few.

Days later the Japanese were proclaiming a great Naval victory in the Coral Sea, though their contradictory behaviour suggested it could not have been the ultimate victory originally mapped out.[4] Parties of Naval Officers arrived at the Mission and questioned the missionaries and local people about the mountains, rivers and jungles of the New Guinea mainland. They descended on the library at Vunapope seeking information and maps and made no secret of the fact that their goal to take Port Moresby, which was vital to the Japanese conquest of Australia, was yet to be achieved. Father Barrow told us that the old-timers in Rabaul were astounded when they heard of the Japanese intention to approach Port Moresby on foot over the formidable Owen Stanley Range. Bold exclamations that the Japs would never make it were heard everywhere.

May passed into June and the last few months of stability and comparative tranquillity had lulled us into a false sense of security. We had become complacent, even careless in some regards as we were soon to find out.

'Get up! Get up! The Commander is here!'

There was much shouting and tramping of heavy boots on the stairs, then soldiers with rifles and fixed bayonets pointing downward surrounded our beds. It was four o'clock in the morning and we were prodded down the stairs in our night clothes and lined up on the lawn. In the half-light we were shocked to see the nuns being treated likewise. The chilly air and our apprehension caused some of us, including me, to shiver as we were formed into groups of four.

'I hope they don't think we're afraid of them,' I whispered to Joyce.

'Don't worry they know darn well we are, look what they're doing now.'

Kit-bags, cases and drawers were dragged downstairs and thrown on the grass; they started hauling out clothing and books and, horror of horrors to many of us, diaries. Books and various papers were put to one side and we noticed that the Japs scarcely glanced at them - probably because they couldn't read English! Whatever they were looking for must have been important to them; mattresses, pillows and cupboards now joined the pile on the lawn. Mary admitted to me that she was relieved to see the nuns were revealed as being hoarders of junk, just as she was and knew me to be. Everything was meticulously examined by the Japs, clothing shaken and the pockets turned out, cottonwool unwound and even toilet rolls unrolled.

While all this activity was keeping the Japanese occupied a rumour started circulating that an Allied invasion was imminent and that we were all being sent away. As this discussion got under way it was received with mixed feelings - after all, if there were to be a landing by our Allies, we all hoped to remain right here. Our talking ceased and the Japs' enthusiasm for their job waned as the temperature began to rise with the morning sun. The Japs took themselves off and left only a skeleton crew in charge of operations.

A few of the girls plucked up enough courage to go to the *benjo*. The bolder ones and those with something to hide made a gesture towards their belongings and, to their surprise and great relief, the guard just nodded and off they went to shred incriminating writings down the outdoor lavatories. I was among those who were not so lucky. My property rested at the foot of a sullen looking character who, unlike his compatriots, ignored the hot sun and stood guard like a true soldier of Nippon. Afraid to arouse his suspicions the four of us just stood and suffered with him until at last, at about 11am, we were told we could leave. I made a gesture towards my belongings and was halted by a muffled grunt; this hostile fellow got out the ubiquitous handkerchief, carefully tied up everything and marched off.

Later that afternoon one of the nuns came hurrying across the lawns and happily handed our diaries and other possessions back to us. The diaries had not been opened. She delivered, as well, an order from the Mother Superior: All written articles of an incriminating nature to be destroyed and no further writings of this kind to be attempted.

We needed no more warning and wrote a letter of apology to the Mother Superior, we had no wish to create any problems for her.

After this we went across to visit Grace, who was very ill in the Convent sick bay with a high temperature and septic throat. She told us that a Japanese doctor had been to see her that morning and, after asking a few questions, made some comment to his aide and left. We had no inkling then that this visit by the Japanese doctor, to our sick colleague, was to be instrumental in saving our lives - the lives of all the Army, Government and Missionary nurses and Kathleen Bignell, prisoners of the Japanese at Vunapope at this time.

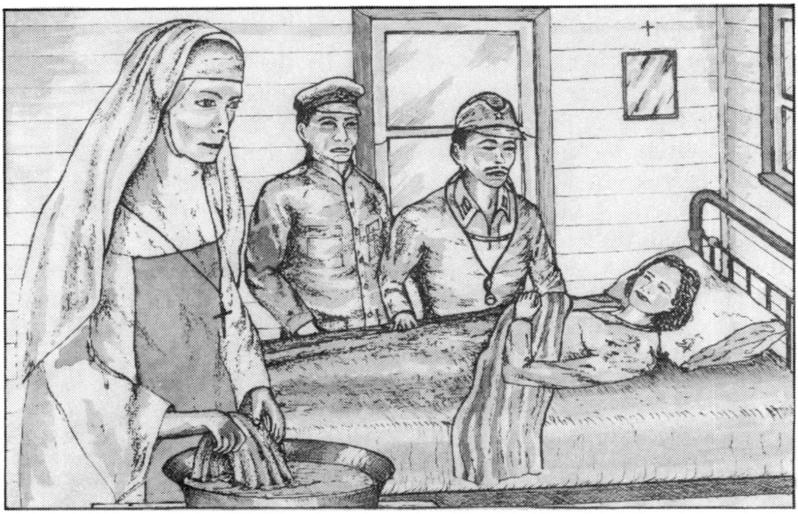

Grace in the Convent sick-bay

As this trouble weary day drew to a close a few of us tried a little diversion and settled down to a game of checkers. A full moon cast a day-like radiance over the Mission grounds and the only disturbance in this strangely peaceful setting was the zooming and buzzing around our ears of copra beetles. Presently in walked Father Barrow not with his usual jaunty air and broad smile; he looked rather distraught and haggard.

'There is no easy way to tell you girls this,' he said, 'today all the men in the camps in Rabaul, apart from the Army officers and a dozen or so civilians kept to do specialised work, were put on a Japanese freighter. They were given no warning and no explanation as to their destination. The ship is named the *Montevideo Maru*. All your doctors were taken away, with the exception of Doctor Watch, and we also lost our two Australian Mission priests. No opportunity to send messages was given. The men just called out and waved as they were being rounded up by the Japs and marched down to the wharf.' Doctor Watch, being South African, seemed to enjoy a position of benevolent neutrality. South Africa was a divided country under two flags, the one British and the other Afrikaner, whose leanings were undeniably pro-German. South Africa joined Britain's cause in World War II after the ruling United party, which was pro-British, won the vote in Parliament by a very slim margin.

We were not geared for such a shock as this and it left us numb with disbelief. Where were so many to be taken? No thought was ever entertained that such a thing could happen and we all silently prayed they would be safe wherever they were headed. Mary's husband, Tom, could not be located among the prisoners in Rabaul. Father Barrow had made constant inquiries as to his whereabouts, but no one came forward with any information, which gave Mary hope that he had escaped with the fortunate ones.

The imprisoned ranks of Lark Force totalled more than eight hundred men and there were well over two hundred civilians and remnants of the New Guinea Volunteer Rifles in the camps. We did not know the exact number but among them were Plantation owners and Plantation managers, senior Civil Administration officers, Public servants, merchants and professional people, and Australian missionaries from all denominations. Most of the civilians had played a role, either small or large, in the development of the Territory since the Mandate was granted. The Norwegian sailors who survived the sinking of the *Herstein* were also among these prisoners.

Thoughts void of all feeling but sorrow followed this heart-wrenching news of our boys as human cargo, but were interrupted by Father Barrow's next comment.

'That Japanese doctor who was prowling around here when you girls were lined up this morning called with one of the officers to see Sister Kruger. After a close examination he found her to be very sick with a high fever. Following a conference between the two Japs the Doctor said, "She will be too much trouble at this stage and being a woman she is of no consequence, so leave her where she is".'

'And,' Father Barrow added emphatically, 'that is the reason why you girls are still here and not on your way with the men.'

Take us away! Why would the Japanese need to take us away from the Mission? It made no sense, we did not consider ourselves to be a threat as prisoners, yet on receipt of this incredible piece of information we no longer felt secure at Vunapope.

We could only describe ourselves as stunned by all this distressing news from Father Barrow and, added to the events of our own day, everything weighed heavily with us. Over a cup of tea Father Barrow informed us of the real reason for the search this morning. The Japanese were worried about the accuracy of recent bombing raids and were searching for evidence of hidden radios.

'It is strange you know, the Japs don't seem to be worried about our heroic coastwatchers - our missionaries in the bush sometimes meet up with them.' To our disappointment he said no more on this subject and we could not draw him out either as we knew any information these days must be kept secret. "Loose lips, sink ships", we had heard so many times when German raiders stalked the seas before the Japanese struck. We were aware that many plantation owners and managers along with Government District and Patrol Officers, all having a wide knowledge of the area, were engaged in this important clandestine work of observing the happenings along the unguarded coastlines and waters of New Guinea and the Solomon Islands. It was one of our coastwatchers, Con Page, a Copra plantation manager on Tabar Island who gave early warning of most of the raids on Rabaul and the approach of the Japanese fleet before invasion.[5]

The piece of news concerning the reason for this morning's search cheered us up a little as we did not think the Japs were worried about anything. Once again our hopes were raised that an Allied invasion and our deliverance might come soon. This day which, oddly enough, ended in optimism was the 22nd of June 1942.

Exactly twelve days after that disturbingly memorable date hordes of Japanese again invaded our sanctuary. We had just come in from a walk to the Mission cemetery when Sugai the *Interpreter* arrived with several Naval officers, one of whom stood out noticeably from his companions. He was tall and looked more southern European than Oriental. With much over emphasised bowing, Sugai introduced him.

'This gentleman is from the House of Mitsubishi. You must obey him,' said Sugai totally ignoring the other officers. As none of us, at this stage, had heard of the House of Mitsubishi this honour was completely lost on us.[6] Before Sugai could give us any instruction this important person addressed us in a well educated English voice.

'Please, just call me Michael.' Speechless gasps greeted this invitation - we were all too astonished to call him anything, much less *Michael*!

The other officers directed us upstairs, which further added to our confusion, and apprehension. When Sugai ordered everything to be taken out of drawers and cupboards, he gave an award winning performance, inflated with bogus authority by Michael's revered presence. Forceps and scissors were confiscated.

'How many blankets have you?' A puzzling question!

Downstairs again, still adopting the same, imperious air, Sugai made an announcement.

'You have been handed over to the Imperial Japanese Navy and these officers will visit you every month.'

We didn't know what to make of this switching of control, but we all agreed that these Naval types looked more civilised than their Army counterparts!

Never did a *month* pass so quickly. The same officers *visited* the very next day and ordered us to pack. Word of our obvious departure from Vunapope soon spread. The Mission nuns appeared with anything these resourceful ladies could lay their hands on, which might be likely to come in handy: clothing, sheets, towels, old fancy dresses, soap, cutlery and several bottles of wine!

Michael stood by eyeing everything.

'You will not need those' he said, spotting mosquito nets. 'You are going to Paradise.'

Paradise! Again we found ourselves speechless by another remark from this man. Alarmed as well as confused, no one could find the courage to ask what was meant by *paradise*.[7]

We dawdled over the packing but could not delay the inevitable for long. Michael told us to say goodbye. Only Father Barrow, the Bishop and the nuns we knew were allowed to be present; we sang *Auld Lang Syne* and *Home Sweet Home* and then took a very tearful farewell. These good people had given us so much comfort and shelter for the past six months we knew we would miss them.

No swaggie of the outback was better equipped than we were that traumatic day when we clambered aboard the waiting lorry clutching cans, bottles, wooden boxes, kit-bags and a few suitcases. Soon we were out along the coast road heading to Rabaul. We passed Raluana Methodist Mission where the native children hailed us; continuing on past sombre Vulcan we pulled in beside a new building near the small Malagunan Mission not far from Rabaul.

Here the scene had changed considerably since we passed this way six months ago. Littering this once beautiful beachfront were untidy huts surrounded by garbage and uprooted trees entangled in barbed wire; newly erected wharves and landing stages jutted out into the sea. This was the once delightful Blue Lagoon area, where swimming parties took tea under the palm trees. Such happy memories were shared by us all, though I must say in the cool of dusk when the Angelus-bell rang out there was always a scramble for cars to make a hasty departure before the mosquitos descended.

Off shore a freighter of about seven thousand tons was anchored, no one spoke as our vehicle started up after refuelling.

The lorry drove off the road a little way further along and came to a halt at the beachfront. Without saying a word the guard jumped down and beckoned us to do likewise. We were watching a landing barge bouncing over the waves towards us.

The young man who approached was somehow refreshingly familiar. His uniform was not so different from that of our own Naval officers and the contrast between the two, as he took over from the Army officer who was escorting us, made the latter look like something out of the jungle.

Formalities were brief and we were waved on in the direction of the barge, now resting on the beach. Vigilantly guarding all our worldly possessions we heaved ourselves aboard.

Heading across the bay the blinding reflection of the sun struck an alien note, shimmering off new tin roofs on the shacks, constructed by the Japs, along the waterfront. The ruins of Rabaul showed up dismally as we got further out in the harbour. Many landmarks were already destroyed, and cherished memories of this once lovely town added to our sadness as we gazed at the green hills in the background. With a last glance at The Mother and ever belching Matupi we rounded the stern and crept into the shadow of the freighter. Smudgy white letters spelt out her name, *Naruto Maru*, and something told me we were going *longwe tumas*.

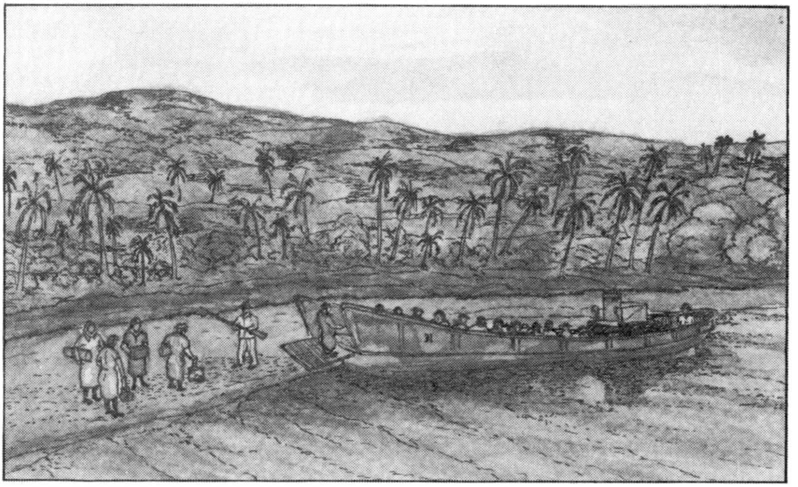

Boarding the barge for departure

5

A SEA VOYAGE

The gangway of the *Naruto Maru* was suspended alongside the hull. It was bobbing up and down in the slight ocean swell and presented a rather daunting sight to us, weighed down as we were, with so much luggage.

'Come on girls, it's not as bad as it seems,' said Kay, swaying alarmingly from side to side as she ventured upwards.

We arrived safely on deck without mishap and stood around confused and bewildered as did the Jap Naval guard. Was this the Japanese way or were the Japs overwhelmed at the appearance of a group of Australian women? After a few minutes of indecision the guard sprang to attention and indicated that he wanted us to line up. There was no roar of the familiar *Tenko*, perhaps that was not part of the Naval vocabulary.

After a while, apparently satisfied that none of us had taken a dive from the gangway on the way up, he uttered his first English words.

'Down there,' he said, unassertively, while pointing to an opening in the deck.

Kay led the way and the rest of us followed. Mugs and bottles tied to bags and swags clanged as they bounced off the steep ladder. One by one we came to rest on the slatted floor of the hold with our pieces of luggage remaining intact. Thankfully, we noticed that the guard had not followed.

'What now?' was asked; no one was ready with an answer.

'I wonder if we will get tea and something to eat when we go up on deck again?' Joyce said. There was a clear answer for us all when the guard appeared at the head of the ladder.

'You stay there.' He used a more authoritative manner this time.

Finally Kay broke the silence which followed the Jap's unexpected command.

'Ladies, welcome to this spacious cabin put at our disposal by the kind Japanese. Ventilation could be better, there is no water, there are no sea views, the beds will be rather uncomfortable and there is only just the remotest possibility that the lights will come on later. The galley is closed for the time being, the cooks have gone ashore for a few beers!'

An inspection of the hold revealed metal rings in the uprights, and the deck was strewn with heaps of straw and dry hay.

'So this is how those horses came to Rabaul. Well if horses can travel down here, we can too. Don't let's forget that the Japs said we looked like horses.'

Surprisingly, no one thought my remark very funny.

Lolling around on our sole possessions in the hold the silence was oppressive. I began to think over our last few months at Vunapope in the sheltered environment of the Convent; the harsh reality of our unenviable state had eluded us. We had no idea now where we would be going or what would happen to us. Imagine assuming, as we had, that we would be accommodated in the cabins of this passenger cargo ship![1]

'I remember reading a book about our convict ancestors. It was mostly about the women, who were transported in the hold of one of those exceptionally small vessels, flying the red and white pennant, under charter to the British Government. The wretched souls barely existed on a diet of bread and water. Many of them died on the journey of course, but ...'

'Well, I wouldn't spurn a piece of dried bread right now,' Whytie interrupted, 'not to mention a few gallons of water. Anyway those women were with their own kind and I think some of them even had their men with them. A few men down here - real men I mean - would boost our morale no end.' I wondered if Whytie's mind had begun to wander.

Such random meandering took over at intervals from the major issues confronting us; namely the reason for our transportation and our destination. And there was, also, an immediate worry spoken of only in whispers.

'Would the Americans be over tomorrow morning?'

Allied attacking raids had been coming fairly regularly of late and down here in the hold it was not a healthy thought. The possibility of such an event, somehow, did not have the same impact when we were up on deck above the waterline!

Increased activity on deck above caused further speculation below. Were we about to sail tonight? There had been few bombing raids at night and it seemed likely that the Japs would leave under cover of darkness. This was the general opinion of the *experts*.

The commotion above increased and there was mortified silence as everyone listened for the drawing up of the gangway and throb of engines. But there was nothing except the stamping about on deck of heavy feet and the murmur of voices - familiar voices. They were speaking ENGLISH! The murmuring and stamping overhead came nearer; long brown legs appeared over the hatchway and clattered down the ladder. Shrieks of joy and relief greeted these astonished men and we all began talking at once. When the din calmed down a little we recognised men from the New Guinea Volunteer Rifles and officers of the 2/22nd Battalion including the Commanding Officer, Colonel Scanlan. A handful of men from the 1st Independent Company of Kavieng and a lone RAAF Intelligence Officer completed a party of sixty.

The great surprise at this reunion was mutual as we had previously met many of the men in Rabaul. They knew we had been evacuated to Vunapope and naturally assumed we would have been left there for the duration of the war. They could add nothing to our information, received from Father Barrow, of the men who had been put aboard the *Montevideo Maru* two weeks ago; many of them were not imprisoned in the Rabaul camp at the time. Perhaps, they said hopefully, we will all be put in the same camp when we reach the end of this voyage. They told us that there were four men kept in Rabaul, who had been assigned to look after the Freezer for the Japs since the beginning, one was the editor of the *Rabaul Times*, Gordon Thomas, and the other three were engineers. Although Noel was an engineer he was not among those left behind, he was on the *Montevideo Maru*.

Another group of civilians were held by the Japs to carry out specialised work. Included in this group was the manager of W R Carpenter's Pondo Copra Plantation, Bill Korn, who had made a dynamic contribution to the Territory, both in New Britain and on the mainland, since his arrival after active duty in the First World War. My mind reflected on the sinking of the *Herstein* and its *copra before people* cargo; now here was this loyal Territorian, as well as the factory manager of Pondo, Albert Evenson, being forced to foster this cherished commodity for the benefit of the Japs. War certainly did change the sum of things.

Mary sought news of her husband; this time directly from the men of the New Guinea Volunteer Rifles who knew him. They had no information about him and Mary placed her only hope in the adage 'no news is good news'.

The men told us about exchange of Japanese prisoners, interned in America and Australia, with our people who had been living in Japan at the outbreak of the war.

'Don't be too hopeful, but we really can't think of any reason why they would want to remove you girls from Vunapope except for exchange purposes.'

Could this be the answer to one of our questions?

About an hour after we had settled a Japanese officer came down and beckoned four of the men to follow him. Again there was a great deal of stamping and general activity overhead; this brought a rise of tension in nerves that had enjoyed a period of relaxation since the arrival of our men. Half an hour went by before a cheerful voice called out a message down the hatchway.

'Everything is under control - you have been warned - we have just been appointed as chefs to the Hotel la Hold.'

Once again the sweeping opinion was that these Naval Japanese seemed to be showing more aptitude for organisation than their Army counterparts. After a while one of the men went along to see what the cooks were up to and his report was very encouraging.

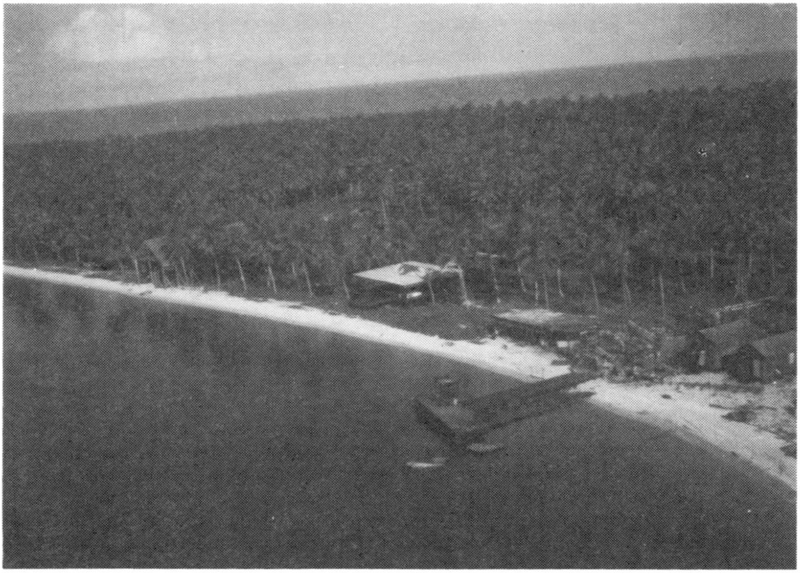

Pondo Copra Plantation

'They are well away above, the Japs have supplied them with wood, coal and a big copper tub to cook sacks of rice. They are setting up lavatories *of a sort* on deck as well.' Without delay we all set to work clearing a space for supper.

When a really savoury aroma drifted through the hatch to the restless hordes below, one of the men paid the supreme compliment.

'Those coves up there must have been cooks in a shearing shed.'

It was well known in outback Queensland before the War that anyone who was able to survive as a shearer's cook had to be *first class*. No one seemed to know how the legend of the cook's status came about. Perhaps it evolved because shearers were a cranky lot and known to have their demands met. Their temperament would have been due to the monotonous, and really strenuous work of shearing vast numbers of sheep in the extreme heat, especially in the days before machines made the job easier. Be that as it may, any cook not coming up to scratch was likely to be dumped in the dam or attacked by the wielder of the tar brush!

Our would-be chefs made a triumphant appearance when slowly down the ladder they came balancing the copper pot carefully between them. They placed it on the deck below and we were served a stew of tinned meat with rice. It was flavoured with bones of indeterminate origin, but was eagerly devoured; biscuits and jam followed, and hearty congratulations to the cooks!

There was little sleep for anyone that night as we caught up with their news of the past six months. A great many of the men had been unsuccessful in attempting to escape and they told us of incredible, distressing experiences in the jungle - much as we had heard from the missionaries - before they were finally captured. Some officers, including the Commander, had surrendered to the Japanese in the hope that leniency would be shown towards the captured troops.

So far the Japanese had scarcely bothered us by their presence. During the evening we went up to the makeshift lavatories on deck which were without doors. No facilities for washing could be seen. A guard was posted on deck by the entrance to the hatch and he didn't bother us either, but sat in a chair with his back to the opening.

Our officers certainly lived up to the Australian reputation for ingenuity. One of them produced an ancient banjo and we joined him humming and singing hill-billy tunes while, yet later, sounds of a harmonica contributed to sentimental recollections of a bush campfire. As the night wore on, the air in the hold became very thick and we crowded *en masse* beneath the open hatchway. When the dawn came a few hardy individuals were playing cards. The face of the cards had undergone many treatments with mercurochrome; the cards themselves had very little shuffle left in them, but they still functioned.

Audible sighs of relief greeted the morning as stiff forms rose from the thin coverings scattered over the slatted floor. There was a unanimous opinion this morning that slats could certainly be improved on as a bed foundation regardless of Pastor Abbott's opinion, expressed at the Mission. We were folding up our bedding and thinking longingly of hot baths and breakfast when a Japanese officer appeared at the top of the hatch and ordered everyone on deck. We were made to stand to attention as a solemn procession, carrying the ashes of the Japanese War dead, came up the gangway. Since this ship was entrusted to transport this sacred item, one thing appeared certain, our destination would be Japan. At the end of the ceremony of the 'handing over of the casket' there was widespread relief when the Japanese officer said we could remain on deck. We stole a look at the sorry state of Rabaul standing out clearly from the deck of the ship, and were left to wonder how it would survive the ravages of war.

Buckets of salt water were provided for washing and our resourceful men found pieces of canvas to screen us. In no time came the announcement: 'Ladies your bath is ready.' We did appreciate that *bath* in salt water, even though we could get no lather out of the soap and our privacy was a bit sketchy.

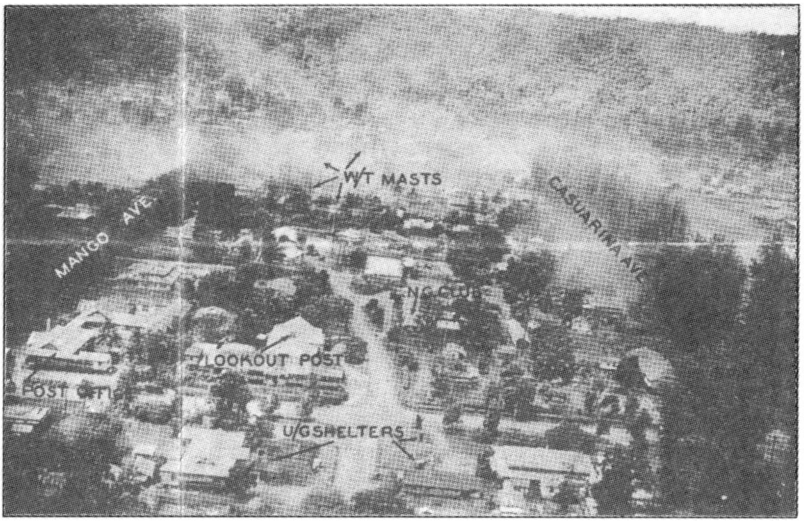

The sorry state of Rabaul

About 10am everyone was ordered below. The air, that had been crisp and fresh above, turned into a blanket of hot wet heat down here in the hold, which was already taking on the smell of a long-closed building. This atmosphere did nothing to help the tension, which instinctively gathered momentum as we listened for any sound that would herald the approach of planes. We prayed that our aircraft would not be over today, and no one among us put voice to that very real possibility of being bombed while battened down below. Such thoughts were obviously better left unspoken. A siren blared.

'That's only a passing ship,' volunteered several of the men at once. Never was the likelihood of a visit by our planes more unwelcome as on that morning of 6th July 1942, which was almost six months to the day since the first Japanese raid on Rabaul.

For the next two hours there was increasing activity on board and around noon when the engines began to throb the hatch cover was slammed shut. This was one of the worst moments of our lives.

'Don't worry,' came the reassurance from the Colonel, 'when we clear the harbour they'll open it up again.' Thankfully he was right and after a few days at sea the constant fear of bombs receded.

The reassuring presence of our men and the more relaxed attitude of the Japanese added to a sense of well-being for us. Could this faintly resemble *a sea voyage*? Boxes were made into small sets of tables and covered with odds and ends; here we played cards and talked of the wonderful time when we would all be free again. Gourmet feasting played a large part in these discussions of the future and we were forced to admit that the men far outstripped the women conjuring up meals of many courses.

One evening Joyce discovered that a bottle of wine she had wrapped in cotton wool was broken. Little was wasted as we sieved the wine into a glass and dried the wool for future use. What better time to open the bottles of wine the nuns had given us before a similar fate should befall the rest of them. A small tot each added a festive touch to the now routine meal of rice and tinned meat stew, and we all drank a toast to the future.

Later we distributed native tobacco leaf which was another gift from the missionaries. While the men enjoyed an after dinner smoke we, the females of the group who were being rather pampered on this trip, cleared away the dishes.

Many officers had been living in unthinkable conditions in bush camps, before being interned in Rabaul a few weeks prior to departure. They suffered bouts of malaria and several had tropical ulcers; the jungle-like atmosphere of the hold was detrimental to their health, particularly to their ulcers. We had some dressings available and were pleased to have quinine for the malarial sufferers. Sailing into the cooler summer of the northern hemisphere, we hoped, would show an improvement in the stifling and almost intolerable conditions below decks.

On the occasions we were allowed on deck we found it reasonably cool. We were travelling with two or three other ships and, although we knew that there was no distinguishing insignia on our vessel to show that prisoners of war were being carried, we felt somewhat safeguarded in convoy. There was a very limited supply of fresh drinking water and we could use only salt water for bathing and washing of clothes. The men said we had sufficient food for about two weeks, due to items they had scrounged before coming on board and supplies the nuns had given us. The Japanese provided rice and bread so I suppose our situation could have been worse.

Australian men have never been considered domesticated and I am sure not even the mothers and wives of these men on board would have credited them with the skill displayed in taking charge of cooking and laundry arrangements. After hauling up buckets of water from the sea they immediately got on with their washing, mostly accompanied by bursts of song and remarks about such chores.

'Your washing isn't Persil white this morning Mrs 'Arris, you'd better switch to Sunlight, just look at this 'ere.'

This seemingly light-hearted patter, interspersed with snatches from *Waltzing Matilda* or *Kiss Me Goodnight Sergeant Major* or other popular wartime ditties, caused passing Japanese to stop and ponder.

'Are you happy because you sing?'

Salt water and soap that could raise no lather was a disastrous combination. One day, when a Japanese officer stopped near the washerman of the day he suggested that a good idea would be to do as they did in the old days at sea and tie the clothes to a rope trailing over the stern. This was said to make the washing whiter than white as it tumbled in the ship's wake. The suggestion was not really appreciated and certainly not acted upon. The hatch cover and nearby wood pile made an excellent drying area for laundry and a favourite or, perhaps I should say, the only seating area.

Just north of the Equator the high black peaks of the Caroline Islands gave us our first sight of land. On the morning of our third day at sea the men came back from their early visit to the upper deck to report that we were travelling alone. Quite possibly the ships in convoy had returned to their base at Truk in the Carolines.

'We are probably considered to be out of the Allied danger zone,' said one of the men. I must say it was a relief to put being bombed at sea into the *not so likely* category. We girls had not really considered a submarine attack and no mention of that *highly likely* possibility was made by the men.

During their internment the officers in the Rabaul camp had worked with the ranks and civilians unloading supplies from Jap ships, and the collection of things acquired was remarkable, though not all were acquired while in the *employ* of the Japs. Our sheltered life at the Mission had not prepared us in becoming self-sufficient as prisoners of war, we were fledglings in this respect. Remembering Father Barrow's comments relating to the exploits of the men at the wharves and a possible connection to the dubious ancestry of some Australians, I could not help thinking that then, as now, necessity was the mother of invention. Hadn't a great many of those transported convicts stolen only in an endeavour to save their families from starvation during insufferable times of famine and cruel oppression?

After supper on the sixth day at sea the men dragged out their swags and laid, as they said, their treasures at our feet. We were astounded at the quantity and variety of the spoils. Spread out on blankets were glass mugs, towels, tubes of toothpaste, soap, toilet paper, *laplaps* (the uniform of the native houseboy, some with the employer's name embroidered on the hem for laundry identification), and, standing apart, was a set of embroidered sheets and a pair of beautiful lace curtains from Manila. These latter, said their owner, came from the Rowse house, which was one of the many homes searched for items to aid survival.

'When I get back I am going to congratulate that lady on her good taste,' he said. I declined the offer of these curtains and accepted a heavy glass beer mug instead. We did not, at this early stage of captivity, appreciate the potential bargaining power of certain goods and under our present circumstances I could not think of any possible use for lace curtains!

Every day now the Japanese officers became more and more relaxed and were happy to acknowledge that our destination was Japan. They, no doubt, felt they had a fair chance of getting home safely.

I asked one of our own officers if he thought these Naval men were not superior to the Army Japanese we had encountered. He thought awhile before replying, being an Army man himself.

'Well, they do seem to be more agreeable. The British taught the Japs ship building and officers of Japan's Navy attended Naval Colleges in Britain, and mastered the English language, so maybe they are.'

In spite of the calm weather and cooler climate, the over-crowded conditions and lack of the most elementary hygiene made life below decks oppressive and almost unbearable, especially during the long nights. I dare not let myself think of Noel and the others on this same journey, crowded as they must have been with over a thousand men in the hold, suffering unthinkable conditions that could never be compared with our own.

Taking advantage of the general tolerance of the Naval Japs, we began going on deck in small numbers during the night. No one bothered us on these occasions and the guard in his chair at the top of the ladder was always asleep or at least pretending to be. One night however there was a terrible commotion. The guard must have really dozed off and his rifle bounced down the ladder just missing the head of a young man of the 1st Independent Company. This man, notorious for his loud snoring, knew nothing of what had happened until he was told in the morning and, naturally, refused to believe it.

On our ninth day at sea we sighted the land of Dai Nippon. On finding out from one of the officers that Dai Nippon actually meant Great Japan, I could only assume that it was Japan's wish to emulate Great Britain. I couldn't think of any other country defined as Great! Only in recent years has Japan claimed to be the Great Empire of Japan, presumably in reference to the *great* Japanese plan of *territorial expansion*.

The *Naruto Maru* rounded the Bozo Peninsula and we were ordered to stay below but, luckily, we were allowed on deck again as we approached the wharf at Yokohama in Tokyo Bay. There was very little in the way of shipping here for such a large port and fussy little lighters were busy unloading freighters as we steamed among them. We came near a German vessel with a very neglected air about her, as though she had been laid up for some considerable time; across her stern was the name, *Ramses*.[2] Unkempt men hung over the rails and turned their binoculars on us as we anchored alongside. They must have got a shock at the sight of eighty odd Australian men and women journeying on a Japanese freighter.

Several men were familiar with the geography of the Tokyo area and pointed out places of interest around the bay. On the peninsula to the right the industrial centre was heavily enveloped in smoke. In contrast, on the other side, the steep slopes of the Bluff, green and tree covered, lay silhouetted against the setting sun. Just on dusk the fishing fleet, gently bobbing with the ocean swell, entered the harbour; a host of striped sails fanning in the breeze added to the illusion that war was a long way from these shores.

Having seen pictures of wartime England and the Continent and now viewing first-hand this seemingly peaceful seaport, we were quite surprised to find no signs of a country at war. There were no warships guarding Tokyo Bay and there seemed to be no blackout restrictions, millions of lights lit the seaboard and the city of Yokohama.

'Looks like Sydney on a summer evening, only the entire harbour here would be lost in just one of the bays in Port Jackson.' This nostalgic remark from one of the officers startled those near and we looked around furtively to see who might be listening. There were no Japanese in sight and I naively assumed they wouldn't be familiar with Sydney Harbour anyway!

'Down below.'

The Japanese officer's voice was quite pleasant. He had come home safely! And, with very mixed feelings, we went below for the last time.

There was no cooking allowed on deck this evening and after a supper of tinned fish and left over rice the smokers enjoyed the last of their tobacco leaf. Tonight there was nothing left to discuss. Apprehension was too apparent to allow for anyone to pretend to be optimistic. The last eight nights down here had been made bearable as the present was pushed into the background; the past with perhaps some embellishments had taken centre stage and the distant future was presented as rosy by our travelling companions. But, when this new day dawned on 16th July 1942, after a long and sleepless night the only thing certain was the present. We were about to be off-loaded in this foreign country of Japan with which Australia was at war and we were prisoners of that war.

'Be ready in an hour.' An officer clambered down the ladder to give this command making no attempt to disguise the cheerfulness of his manner. He suggested that in the meantime we could *make tea*.

Over a breakfast of black tea and dry bread, the men repeated what they had said previously about the possibility of nurses being exchanged. We received last minute messages from them for relatives and friends at home and rolled up our swags. It was time to go above.

This morning the German crew on the deck of the freighter would be really puzzled as to where this motley crowd, emerging from the hold, had come from, and indeed, could possibly be going.

A close-up would have revealed a large group of people, with tins and bottles and bags hanging from them, in various forms of dress and undress (a few men were draped in *laplaps*). We thought we looked much the same as the natives in New Guinea going home to their grass huts after a days work on the plantation.

A small, black-coated man arrived with a retinue of six bureaucrats in white uniforms, heavily trimmed with gold braid. He introduced himself as an inspector from the Foreign Office, but to all of us then, and ever after, he was referred to as the Undertaker. He looked us over and, as we had always observed on these occasions, appeared undecided what to do next. While consulting his list he indicated, by waving his hands, that we were to line up. This was achieved with some preciseness, thanks to our officers.

The Undertaker began to count us by walking down the line and pointing at each one with his index finger; he kept referring to his list and carried on like this several times. The men at the head of the line started to fidget and a remark, somewhat louder than a whisper, issued from one of them.

'The silly bastards can't count in their own country either.'

Thankfully there was no reaction from the Undertaker. Either he did not hear or did not understand what had been said, and those of us who did heaved a sigh of relief. When he was satisfied that none of his charges had escaped, he separated us from the men.

'Hurry!' he said.

For the second time within a few months we parted from our protectors and friends and once more we were left to wonder if we would be seeing our men again.

Ashore the eighteen of us were herded into the Customs Shed. The seedy looking men lounging against the walls inside showed no surprise at the sight of the scruffy bunch of females before them. Later, when we talked about their indifferent attitude, we thought there was a strong possibility they might have been drugged, though we could not think why.

After we were hurriedly searched for cigarettes and books we were bundled into a strange closed-in truck waiting on the wharf. In Australia it would be referred to as a *Black Maria*.

6

THE BUND HOTEL

Few words were spoken during the brief journey from Yokohama's wharf area. Our apprehension was by no means diminished when we stopped in front of a solid two-storey building. Large letters in English above the front entrance told us that this was the Bund Hotel.

The Undertaker ushered our party inside and drafted us in twos and threes into various bedrooms. After having lead a dormitory life for so long there was much whispering as to what might be in store for us in this establishment. We deposited our luggage in the rooms and the consensus was that we should keep together as much as possible. We thought it must have been for no good purpose that we were brought here, but we were determined not to allow our fears to get the better of us.

The Bund Hotel in pre-war days had been a modest tourist class hotel for Western visitors. It was not in any way a Japanese establishment, even to inexperienced travellers like ourselves, whose information was only second-hand regarding accommodation in Japan. The first place we all needed was the bathroom, and here, too, everything was as it would have been in an ordinary hotel in Australia. It was truly marvellous to be rid of the grime of nine days living below decks and nine days of rudimentary washing in salt water, although the water in this Japanese hotel could raise no lather in the soap, either. Joyce, Lik and I decided it would be best to hoard the soap given us by the nuns and use it only if absolutely necessary.

The little round proprietress of the Bund, Mrs Saito, spoke English quite well and wasted no time in telling us where we stood in a most frank and most un-Japanese manner. We had the honour to be installed in her hotel through the goodness of her heart.

'I am not a Christian,' she said 'but I have God in my heart. You can stay here because you have nowhere else to go - no one would have you!'

We were fast gaining the impression that the Japanese were not sure what to do with us and this statement of Mrs Saito's supported our theory.

Mrs Saito's goodness of heart soon revealed itself in a semi-starvation diet, otherwise we were ignored and free to roam about the hotel. It appeared that all the guests were Japanese. We often discussed what overseas visitors to Japan before the war would have thought about these lodgings, and we wondered what fate had befallen alien occupants at the time of Japan's surprise entrance into war.

Obnoxious smells blew in through the windows and doors. Sewer smells mingled with those from the decaying hotel garbage outside; but overriding all of these was the smell wafting in from the green vegetable patch near by. We did not recognise this odour at the time because, quite understandably, we didn't associate it with gardening. We were to learn, much later, that the fertiliser for these crops came from the natural discharges of the human body, and when the shock settled we wondered what precautions were taken against disease from human carriers.

Added to this medley of smells were the nauseating perfumes worn by both sexes of Japanese, and I could understand why it was little wonder they frequently walked about wearing nose and mouth masks.

Rats and mosquitoes constituted a contrast in the livestock of the Bund; the rats were without doubt the biggest and liveliest any of us had ever seen and we were quite scared of them. They were just as much at home gambolling around inside the building as they were outside and no normal cat bent on self-preservation would have confronted any of them. Cats here were conspicuous by their absence!

Children were numerous and most of them were very young. Whether they belonged to guests or whether their parents were employed at the hotel was difficult to ascertain since everyone seemed to be on the same social level. At night these youngsters fell asleep wherever they happened to be, in the lounge, on the stairs, even on the floor in the corridors. They cried miserably when attacked by hordes of mosquitoes, and we were upset to see such neglect.

'So much for Michael's *paradise*,' I said to Joyce and Lik. 'Where would we be now without our nets?' From what we had seen so far there were none in use at the Bund Hotel.

Not long after our arrival a small spritely American woman

of advancing years introduced herself. She had been brought to Japan three weeks previously on a Japanese warship from her home on Attu, an island in the Aleutian Islands group.

'My name is Etta Jones,' she said with a friendly smile.

Gradually we learnt that her husband had been employed by the United States Government as a meteorologist and was executed by the Japanese after the capture of Attu on June the 15th. Judging by her present condition Mrs Jones must have been badly treated, but all she said at this period about her ordeal was that she had been brought to Yokohama and given medical treatment.

'In deference to my grey hairs I suppose.' Later, when we brought up the subject of exchange with Mrs Jones she was dispassionate, but she did add that an exchange ship was out in the harbour right now.

A few days later officials arrived to take control of us; their crisp, white uniforms were appropriately adorned.

'You have been handed over by the Navy to the police of the Foreign Office,' announced an officer complete with pips on his shoulders and a sword swinging by his side. He informed us that Mrs Jones was to 'officially' join our party, increasing our number to nineteen.

During the days that followed this hand over the Police officers made frequent visits to the Bund and were always very polite. They talked of everything from their family troubles to how the disastrous earthquake of 1923 wrought such terrible havoc in Tokyo and Yokohama that the two cities had to be rebuilt. We were told how the hard-working Japanese engineers not only cleverly got the industries back to normal but, at the same time, reclaimed a large area of land along the waterfront. Reconstruction work took a long time and it was hard to believe the cost was estimated at five hundred million pounds.[1]

Then we were told of the typhoons that each year ruined crops, flattened houses and sunk ships. These tropical typhoons originate over oceans, where there is plenty of moisture and little resistance to wind, in regions of the sea where the trade winds meet the Equatorial doldrums. The wind velocity often reached over one hundred and fifty kilometres per hour and as the Pacific typhoons usually travel northerly, towards the pole, these scattered little islands of Japan are right in their path. It seemed to us from these alarming revelations that this country and its people did not enjoy much tranquillity and that these calamities could sooner or later interfere with the progress of the war; we certainly hoped nothing disastrous would happen in our vicinity.

Another talk by the informative police was about fire which without a doubt seemed to have been the worst scourge of all. During the 1923 earthquake more than one hundred and forty thousand people were killed, many by the subsequent fires which destroyed most of Tokyo and Yokohama when the fragile homes burnt to ashes. Homes were built of flimsy material to withstand many minor quakes, which occurred nearly everyday somewhere in Japan. Before the days of electricity, our lecturer went on, frail paper lanterns and open fire burners were the only source of light and heating and disastrous fires were a frequent occurrence. The fires were known as the *Flowers of Tokyo* and I could not believe such a lyrical name for such horrific disasters.

Lookout posts were established all over the city. Not wishing to appear facetious no one asked if these were erected to enable the people to admire the *Flowers of Tokyo* or to warn of their occurrence. However, the story of calamity went on, when electricity was eventually laid on it was so badly installed by a Foreign Power - Great Britain no doubt - that the rats nibbled the wires. And the *Flowers* continued to flourish.

Almost three years later I recalled this lecture as the greater part of Tokyo was burning, though the *Flowers* that night had nothing to do with faulty electrical wiring, or rats.

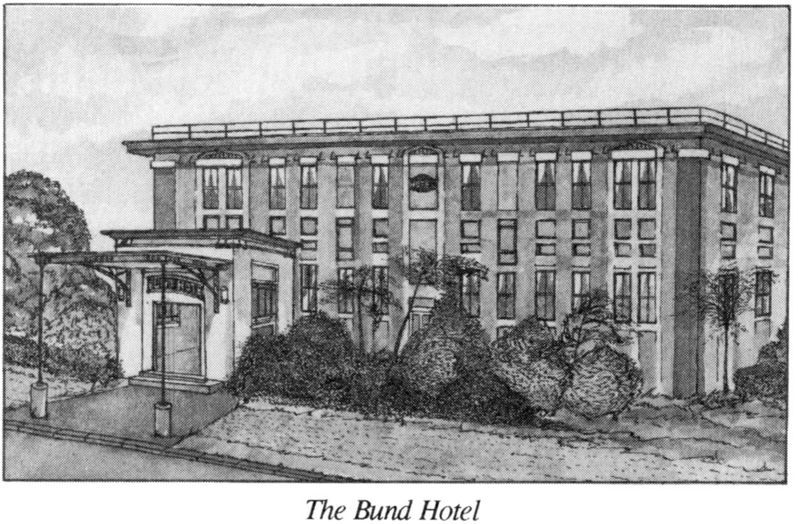

The Bund Hotel

Various other members of the Foreign Office visited us daily. They, also, bombarded us with the most irrelevant questions:

'Are you married?' 'How many children have you?' 'How old are you?' 'Why aren't you married?'

They would not believe we could be in our late twenties and early thirties and not be married. By the time we had finished our training and gained experience, before venturing overseas, the years do not stand still; and the Army girls could not enlist for overseas duty before the age of twenty-five.

'Why? Why?' They kept on asking us, until one day Whytie became irritated.

'Well! The answer is simple if you really must know. *We just haven't had time*.'

The flat roof of the Bund Hotel was out of bounds to us but during the afternoons, when everyone seemed to retire for a siesta, we climbed the stairs to view the city of Yokohama and Tokyo Bay. There was very little shipping here but further around the harbour, almost out of sight, we saw not one but two black ships with big white crosses on the hull. The exchange ships! After our initial burst of excitement we were awe-struck. Surely what our recent travelling companions had said about exchange would soon be a reality.

At the north end of the bay, just behind the hotel lay the Bluff area mentioned by the men. The airy slopes were covered with vegetable gardens, but had been scattered in the past with homes of foreigners living in Japan. At the top was a signal station and a building that was probably some sort of look-out. At the bottom of the gardens stood a large two storey building from which flew the Tricolour; this caused some debate among us. Could there be a French Consul or his representative in residence in a country at war with France? Remembering how the Japs had quickly advanced on Singapore, through Malaya, from bases in French Indo-China, Joyce suggested that the *puppet* Vichy Government of France, which had collaborated with the Germans, was favourable towards the aims of Japan. A representative of the Vichy Government, not the Free French Government, was no doubt occupying the French Consulate.[2]

A few evenings later our guard escorted us downstairs to the Bund's tiny garden. Outside, a squalid neighbourhood of small shops and many smells was revealed. People lived above the shops and washing fluttered from poles jutting from the rooftops. From the many passers-by clip-clopping of *geta* (the traditional Japanese footwear) resounded off the pavements.

The next evening, when we were walking around in the

garden again, a European woman paused by the fence and asked if we were going on the exchange ship. She told us that she was and we said we hoped to see her on board. It was strange speaking to someone *outside* like this, but the encounter left us walking on air. After watching the most powerful searchlight we had ever seen sweep the skies we went indoors to examine our wardrobe, in case of a hurried departure. I am somewhat disappointed to say we were still in our salad days, green in judgement. Although, in the one respect concerning our rationale for being lodged in this hotel in the first instance, I must say we were exceedingly grateful for what was a conceivably, wrong *green judgement*.

There was nothing we could do at the Bund Hotel apart from walk around. One afternoon a few of the girls and I were wandering aimlessly about the corridors when we were stopped suddenly at the sight of Mrs Saito with nothing on. She was vigorously towelling herself while carrying on an animated conversation with a man taking a bath. There was no pause in their discussion nor any notice taken of our presence. We laughed over this in our own chats later, and were to learn that this was not an unusual spectacle. We came to the conclusion that we had discovered more about the Japanese in the past few days than we had in the past six months.

After our first week in Japan ended several European men and women arrived. We were not allowed to contact them and to make it difficult they were housed in an inaccessible wing of the building. We were told that they were missionaries in transit - we felt certain they would be boarding the White Cross ships.

Those beautiful black ships in the harbour were a source of endless discussion. Expectations rose when we were instructed to go to other rooms in the hotel to be inspected by a doctor. This was to be a health clearance required by the shipping line, we were sure. The room where the doctor was waiting was large and opened directly onto the street. The police who brought us here made no move to leave, nor did the doctor order them to do so, but he did tell us rather sharply to remove our clothes. He got on with his very cursory examination while we still clutched the odd garment. Not one of the passers-by in the street even glanced in our direction; the police carried on talking among themselves, as if there was nothing unusual about what we considered a blatant public examination by the doctor. As time went by we learnt that nudity is totally acceptable in Japan and that there is none of the rather false modesty of other nations prevailing in this paradoxical Land of the Rising Sun.[3]

We waited in anticipation of exchange while time passed

monotonously. Mrs Saito hired out her large dining room for social occasions and on one of these evenings, at a distance, we watched what seemed somewhat like a Victorian drawing-room recital, the exception being that all in attendance were called upon to perform.

This night as each participant did his bit - they were all male performers - we became master critics. To Western ears Oriental music is shrill and painful to sight and hearing. The entertainment went on for hours, halted occasionally by the drinking of *sake* and the not very edifying sight of food being shovelled into the mouth with chopsticks. The performance found us filled with nostalgia for the inspiring *sing sings* of the happy, New Guinea people.

In the vestibule of the Bund Hotel there was a mass of flourishing greenery which was most attractive and complimented the outside garden. The Japanese have sometimes been described as the world's best gardeners which could be true. A traditional Japanese garden is said to make a statement symbolising the beauty of nature. Japanese parks feature artificial hills with cascading streams flowing into ponds; narrow arched foot-bridges cross the streams in a time-honoured portrayal of the countryside.

Each morning an old Japanese woman arrived to water the plants in the vestibule and her method seemed so odd as to be primeval. She brought a container of water with her and, by means of a small scoop, filled her mouth with the water and squirted it over the plants. The procedure took some time but she continued in this way until all the plants were nicely sprayed with moisture. This was our first experience as to how the Japanese approach a simple, menial task in a complicated, solemn manner.

Among the greenery in the entrance were receptacles for discarded newspapers and in one of them I was surprised, and excited, to see an English heading, *Japan Times*, a daily Japanese newspaper printed in English. The glaring headlines of this paper dated May this year were all about Japan's glorious victory over the Americans in the Coral Sea and the sinking by the Japs of *Lexington*, the American aircraft carrier. No mention of their own country's losses and the fact that the Japanese were thwarted by this great sea battle and not able to continue in the conquest of Port Moresby and thence also, of Australia.

Mrs Saito, with God in her heart but hatred in her mind, cut our food rations daily, but we were becoming conditioned to eating less and less as the uncertain time passed. The bar at the hotel was being used as a storeroom for vegetables and as we passed here on our way outside we helped ourselves to carrots, onions and anything not too obvious as to draw attention. Had we known then the medium in which these crops were grown we would have been horrified. There was still a great deal more to learn about the Japanese - and ourselves.

There was no avoiding the crazy lectures imposed on us by our new masters from the Foreign Office each time they visited; on one such day they decided to make us the equal of Japanese men. The idea was quite beyond comprehension and seemed pointless. They started by telling us that in Australia women were *above* men and illustrated this by making our mark on a wall and, five inches *lower*, making another, to show where our men were in relation to us. Barely suppressed giggles greeted this demonstration; we had not realised Australian men were so hen-pecked. Then the position was reversed showing the status of Japanese women *lower* than Japanese men. However, as a special concession since we were *visitors* to Japan, they would make us the *equal* of Japanese men!

Anticipation of exchange ran high and any fuel that could fire optimism was ignited. In our discussion about the significance of the curious honour, or dishonour, bestowed on us *visitors* was a word that caught everyone's attention. Yet, as our second week at the Bund Hotel was coming to an end we were bewildered by Mrs Saito's increasing hostility towards us.

'I do not like policemen around my hotel. You will be moved to a place near the sea, but it is not nice like here.'

By now we knew that one should not take much notice of anything these crazy people did or said, yet confusion greeted Mrs Saito's offhand suggestion of a move. Surely we would not be shifted somewhere else when we were about to leave the country. If anything, we decided it would merely be a temporary move before being dispatched. Nevertheless, her disclosure left us unsettled and we patrolled the corridors of the hotel for the rest of the morning hoping to catch a glimpse of the missionaries, seen previously but housed in another wing.

There was no sign of the missionaries anywhere. And when we climbed up to the roof of the Bund that afternoon, there was no sign of White Cross ships either!

7

YOKOHAMA YACHT CLUB

The subtle warning given us by Mrs Saito proved correct and again we found ourselves travelling another short journey along the waterfront in the *Black Maria*. We were off-loaded at the Yokohama Yacht Club. First a hotel now a boating club, but there was really only one thought on our minds: How long were we to be here? We were by the sea as Mrs Saito had said, which kept spirits high and raised our hopes somewhat. The Yacht Club was enclosed by a high wall, but we were confident we would be able to find a way to keep a lookout for White Cross ships.

The Yokohama Yacht Club was a two-storey building. A long room upstairs was partitioned off at each end, one end being a smoking room, the other a ladies room, and in each of these small areas was an open fireplace to keep the members warm in the cold winter months. We were to sleep in this dormitory-like atmosphere. Downstairs a boarded-up archway sealed off some of that area from us, while the remaining part was taken up with showers, toilets and a very large white tiled bath about six feet long by four feet wide and just as deep. This was obviously a communal bath tailored to Japanese custom, yet there was no evidence in the rest of the building to indicate that this Club was in any manner anything other than a *European* Club.

While examining the room like a team of detectives we came across the names of several of our recent shipmates on the inside wall of a small cupboard. Suddenly, Grace, who was near the partition, held up her hand.

'There are men talking in there and they are Australians!' she whispered excitedly.

‘We can’t do anything about contacting them now’ Joyce suggested, ‘the guard might be with them.’

We went back upstairs and waited patiently until we were sure that all the Japs in the vicinity were having their meal. Two of the girls acted as sentries while the rest of us covered the wide deck immediately above the rooms below, where the men were. Their guard was still with them, so we just talked as loud as we could amongst ourselves and hoped they would be able to hear our voices through the many cracks in the wooden flooring.

‘We hope we’ll be able to come out here in the sun again soon.’ This last trivial broadcast rang out before our own guard hustled us inside.

The next morning proved rewarding. Our guard arrived with a companion and we watched them settle down in deep concentration over the game of *Go*. This game is much loved by the Japanese and has been played in the East for thousands of years. It was obvious that this guard was a *Go* addict which meant little attention would be paid to us as he became further involved in the game; the one track mind of the Japanese had become familiar to us now. The opponents become engrossed in this complicated game, with its simple objective to capture more territory on the chequered board than one’s adversary.

The men below were outside the building and when they heard us above a few of them casually moved under our verandah. We let them do all the talking and a note was pushed up between the floorboards. Ongoing communication with the men would be difficult but it was a great comfort to us to know they were nearby. There were eight men in their group. All the officers had been brought here on the day we disembarked; the next morning these eight were separated from the rest for what seemed no apparent reason and told that their comrades were being sent to the big prison camp of Zentsuji on the island of Shikoku, which was across the Inland Sea. Could this be where Noel and the rest of the men on the *Montevideo Maru* were taken?

The Club was proving to be a pleasant surprise. During the first few days our meals were pleasing, containing an abundance of rice served with fish and vegetables, meat and bread. Hopes once again soared. We thought this VIP treatment surely meant that we would soon be exchanged and could give a favourable report back home of internment in Japan. The boys downstairs supported this view, especially as we were civilian nurses and the Army girls non-combatants. The boys held no hope for themselves, combatants were never freed once taken into captivity.

Several pre-war employees of the Club appeared to be still working here. We assumed that they had been taken over by the Foreign Office along with the Club. The prominent two were Fujita, who was the Chef and lost no time in letting us know that he was responsible for our food, and Kimura, who appeared to have been and still to be the head boy or steward.

Kimura lived with his wife and young children in a small house at the rear just near the Club's swimming pool. He proudly introduced his very pretty wife to us. She looked like the classic picture of Japanese womanhood in her *kimono*; the *kimono* was very flattering to the figure, covering flat bottoms and willowy legs. It seemed a pity that Japanese women did not always favour their national costume. In Western dress, their legs seemed to be suspended from the waist as they walked and, like a badly put together doll, fall shapelessly to the ankles.

Presiding covetously over the kitchen was Fujita San - this was how we were to address him. He was a spritely old Japanese and the nearest approach to our alleged ancestors that one could ever wish to see. His wrinkled face was like a dried up prune from which two slender beads glittered. From the back he looked pure chimpanzee; his large ears protruded on either side of his head and his arms, to the elbows, stuck straight out from his shoulders. To complete the picture, all he needed as he tottered around in his *geta* was a fur coat. The *geta*, the clumsy, thonged wooden shoe, worn by all Japanese for any occasion seemed to me to be the cause of this tottering gait, especially when the sole came in varying heights and styles.

Fuji - we had no intention of calling him anything else - made no secret of his dislike for us and in his presence we kept a certain wariness. He had a brand of Pidgin *English* which was exclusively his own. No other Japanese we'd encountered had ever used Pidgin, though some used very odd English. Fuji had once been a seaman and there was no doubt that this was where he picked up this useful jargon. We had no difficultly understanding him, nor he us.

As the days passed the guards became bored with their daily routine and began visiting each other; the one from below decks coming up for tea or to have a game of *Go* with his counterpart. At other times the sentry below was tempted to the wall on the seafront, where on sunny days the odd fisherman was always to be found. Yokohama was an important fishing village long before it grew into a seaport and its community clung steadfastly to the old ways. As the habits of our guardians developed into a more or less set pattern our chances of communication with the men became almost risk free, though we did have to keep a watchful eye out for Fuji, who was always on the prowl and of course Kimura, too, who was both suave and sly.

We were gradually getting to know Kimura better and trusting him less. He spoke English well and appeared a stylish young man wearing what appeared to be a different suit every day. Perhaps the members of this Club had been very generous with money, presents of clothing or both, or had he helped himself to the contents of the lockers downstairs?

One day an official in the white summer uniform of the Foreign Office arrived. We were all out on the deck, about to set up the broadcast for the boys, when Mrs Bignell spotted him getting out of his car. She raised the alarm and as casually as possible we reached the inside as he was coming up the steps. This was not one of the men who had visited the Bund. He appeared more businesslike than the others and politely inquired about our health. He summoned Kay and told her she was to be in charge, since she was the most senior of the nurses. We were to be allotted duties in connection with household and other daily chores, needless to say he meant that we were to be servants to the Jap guards and others at the Club. He left abruptly without the customary lecture, which was a relief.

An appreciative bonus came our way when we were allowed to have the use of the small, but well stacked library, which had previously been kept locked. Discreet inquiries received no clear answers from Kimura as to who was in charge of this international Club, but we established from various notices in the library that there was once a membership of two hundred. What was more interesting to us were the distinctive menus, and general descriptions of parties held here in the evenings. This must have been a delightful Club with frequent dinners and dances celebrating Christmas and other festive occasions as well as the regular aquatic sports. We found this Western style entertainment difficult to visualise in a Japanese city.

The guards, who were in charge of us at the Club, were attached to the Foreign Office and were known as Junsa. At times they were particularly bored on duty and sought, with some success, the opportunity to practice their English on us.

'Is this your husband?' the Junsa inquired of Whytie, on seeing a picture of what surely must have been the ugliest man in the United States stuck on the wall. Whytie had taken an interesting article from the *Times Magazine* and a picture of this man was included on the same page. After an irate outburst from Whytie the Junsa settled down to a talking session which began with another outrageous question. 'Are you a virgin?' Following a further outburst the discussion changed, rather incongruously, to Shirley Temple; this little curly haired lady was apparently a hot favourite with the Japs of all ages. Looking through the *Times Magazine* the Junsa's attention was caught by a bold, eye-catching advertisement which depicted the problem of body odour. The Junsa followed the pictures down the page with his finger, as a small child would, and when he came to the end where the girl and the hero were embracing he yelled in Japanese, *dame dame*, an expression of disapproval, followed by *baka*, meaning silly.

The Japanese knowledge of the Western world was mostly based on America, a country for which they appeared, strangely enough, to have a latent admiration clearly mingled with envy and awe. Their English was full of American words: cans, cowboys, cinemas, *Roosevelto*, *New Yorko* and Washington DC - with familiar words they oft times added an 'o'. The only thing they seemed to know about Australia was Sydney Harbour and, of course, the much maligned *White Australia* policy, which appeared to be a very sore point with them.

We viewed with interest what we considered a contradiction of standards. The Japs declared it was their sole aim in this war to free the Asian and Pacific peoples of their white oppressors while, at the same time, they would become all powerful in an *Asia for the Asians* situation. The restriction of immigrants or so called *White Australia* policy came into focus in Australia as far back as the middle of the last century. In light of a past radical policy in Japan, which isolated the country for two hundred and fifty years from of the vagaries of foreign influence, we did not understand such a contentious viewpoint. In 1901 the Australian Labour Party introduced The Immigration Restriction Act to limit excessive numbers of foreigners from entering Australia; it was seen in those days as the only way to maintain the existing standard of wages and jobs and to prevent an obvious threat to the country's workforce.[1]

The Junsas' interest in England centred around the King (whose name was Georgie) and that distant newcomer who caused dissent, Mrs Simpson. We found these English language sessions amusing and taught them to say: *God save the King*; but when they walked around blazonly reiterating the enemy's oath of allegiance we hastened to divert them by asking about their homes and families. These guards were not unfriendly, merely lonely like some of the very young, provincial Japs we'd encountered at Vunapope.

The day of August the 20th was bright and sunny and those of us not engaged in kitchen and cleaning chores were out on the verandah. There seemed to be little hope of communication with our friends this morning, the guard with them was unusually talkative and waving his hands about excitedly. Several of the girls settled down to read in the sun. The rest of us strolled around the deck, which was surrounded by the seven foot high wall, previously mentioned, fortunately though there were many peep-holes in it. Suddenly Joyce, who was looking towards the harbour gave a shriek and we all rushed forward.

'It's the black ships!' Joyce said in a loud whisper, then remembering the guard she pointed downwards.

We were certain that the men would have heard more about these exchange ships and would have some information for us. Our hopes were soaring, but impatience mounted as the Junsa below remained close to his charges. During the rest of the morning the lookouts drew us like a magnet to view these two ships. We could see no sign of life on board, but the White Crosses stood out like talisman against the black background of the hull. At long last the Junsa went off to join his cronies on the waterfront and not long after came the call we were waiting to hear.

'Go ahead, all's clear.' Could an invitation have been more welcome? We listened almost without interruption while first one and then another told what he had heard from the guard this morning.

The White Cross ships brought home to Japan many Japanese who had been interned in America and Australia - the exchange had taken place in Lorenzo Marques, on the south-east coast of Africa. There were likely to be further exchanges as long as there were Japs still interned anywhere where they could be repatriated. However, the Junsa could give them no information about internees who might be likely to be exchanged from Japan.

'Perhaps that will come later,' the men said hopefully.

The return of the Japanese prisoners of war marked a turning point for us. The last few promising weeks of adequate food and reasonable treatment ended when the grievances of the exchange prisoners were aired in the press.

A few days later, several people whom Fuji referred to as *big men* arrived from the Foreign Office. The Junsa lined us up and told us to perform the usual bow of respect and thank the kind gentleman! Kay was called forward and ordered to read the front page of the *Japan Times*. The exceedingly prominent headlines had been heavily underlined and as Kay read we were astounded by the trivia. The attitude expressed towards America was beyond doubt venomous and the whole article remarkably childish. Australia, it read, was just a poor relation of Britain who had sold out to the Americans and had now become the forty-ninth state of America.

In Australia, the report went on to say, the camp at Hay was fairly agreeable though in the desert. This locality upset the Japanese, who were not used to such heat and, worst of all, were forced to eat mutton three times a day without rice. One could not expect too much refinement from the Australians of course on account of their convict background. This was too much for some of the girls who started to giggle, the rest of us tried to cover up by coughing. Worse was to come and Kay paused for a few moments trying to quell the interruption. The Japanese looked puzzled.

The revelations continued. Australian women when quite young become very fat and look like sheep. The men had such big feet they had to back up to a door to knock. In America the unfortunate Japanese internees were housed in stables. They were given turkey and cranberry sauce for dinner last Christmas but, like all American food, it contained no pickles. As a result of this lack in their diet many Japanese died of Vexation! The British were let off with less criticism than the other Allies, they merely humiliated a high-ranking Japanese official by making him do his own laundry. This insult reduced his subordinates to tears, yet nothing was said which suggested there might have been an offer, by them, to do this chore for their sadly deflated superior.

After Kay had come to the end of this extraordinary report we were told to "thank the kind gentlemen who were giving us a vacation by the sea".

My thoughts were dwelling on his definition of our position. Vacation was a word with a nice impermanent ring about it. Most of us were, however, losing faith in the meaning of any words uttered by the Japanese. At the Bund Hotel words had been used to the effect that we were *sitting on the fence* and we clutched at this indecision of the Japs. We were fast gaining the opinion that with the absence of choice we had fallen off on the wrong side and a journey downhill was beginning.

When the story of 'living in stables' came up later that day we asked Mrs Jones, our American friend, if she thought this could be the truth.

'They'd be lucky if that were so. Those stables are in America's most famous racecourse and they would have every amenity,' she said with an indignation foreign to her usual placid attitude. 'I can tell you, that the internees would be living in such comfort, and probably luxury, that very few Japanese would be likely to know.'

The editor of the *Japan Times* was Japanese. Apparently the paper was read by most foreigners in Japan, which was just as well because if the paper's readers reiterated many of the articles outside Japan no one would have believed them. One thing we found very hard to reconcile was why large feet would force men to back up to a door in order to knock!

The days towards the end of August were proving a sad time for us. The first disappointment happened as soon as we got to the lookout on the deck.

'They've gone!' a chorus announced. No one had to ask what this meant; the exchange ships were not in the harbour. Later that day the men confirmed that they too had heard the news.

'Don't give up hope they will be back, we have heard that there are quite a number of prisoners still likely to be exchanged.'

Later, we enjoyed a laugh with them about the remarks in the *Japan Times*; they, too, had seen a copy of the paper airing the complaints of the returned prisoners of war.

There was more bad news.

'We are leaving today,' came the message from below. 'We have been told that we are to broadcast to Australia this afternoon. Please listen carefully, we have told the Japanese that we will send messages to our families and that is all.'

Fortunately we were able to be out on deck and heard the messages broadcast from start to finish. Having the final say a newly married officer brought the one-sided talks of assurances, advice and affection to an end.

'Be careful Gwen, on that new bicycle of yours - you know how dangerous the traffic is in Sydney.' The poignant irony of his message made it the saddest of all.

Soon after the officers departed, we were ordered to clean up the room downstairs where they had been detained. Other visitors were expected and the idea of more company cheered us quite a bit. The Junsa would give no further information regarding the anticipated arrival.

There were padlocked cupboards in this part of the building, with names on them, obviously holding the property of members of the Club. The scrubbing and cleaning was of the members' change-room and became almost recreational without the presence of the Junsa and old Fuji. We forgot our loneliness as we made pleasant conversation about the good times they must have enjoyed in pre-war days. We pictured them coming back after a boat race discussing the events of the afternoon, no doubt with the wisdom of hindsight. In the reliving of the race there would always be someone convinced that an unwise decision, perhaps a starboard tack taken too late leaving the wind sit in the shoulder of the sail, was when the race was lost. After a hot shower to remove the salt and sweat of the struggle we visualised them plunging into the communal bath next door. Refreshed, they would relax over a drink only to wait the passing of another week to take up the never-ending challenge.

A few days later the awaited guests settled into their shipshape premises. The barricade between the bathroom and their room was of course still there but, as before, we lost no time in making illicit contact with them. The new arrivals were women, American and English missionaries, and some of them were nuns.

Our new neighbours thought they were going to Tokyo and had no knowledge of exchange plans, relating to them, although their anticipation was high. Some of their members had come from China and had brought their own beds with them. A Japanese nun, who was the first we had seen, brought them food. We learnt that there were missionaries of many denominations in Japan who had come here when the new and reformed government abandoned the two century old policy of seclusion, a policy that was designed for the very purpose of keeping Christianity out. Our missionary neighbours left a few nights later and when they called out goodbye they confirmed their destination was Tokyo.

The days passed slowly now. In front of the Club there was a large area of vacant land and on two or three occasions we had noticed two men riding horses around. We began to refer to them by female names - Gert and Nance - so as not to arouse any suspicions if Fuji or the Junsa heard us discussing them. Nance was young with blond curly hair and looked very smart in his riding outfit. Gert was middle-aged, thickset and not very tall, and one morning when he was alone he raised his hand and called out to us as we walked beside the fence. We thought we detected an Irish accent. Later we learnt that Nance was the German Consul's son. Gert would not recognise us when Nance was with him!

At the end of October winter came to the northern hemisphere and we were in no way fortified to combat the cold weather. In the distance we noticed for the first time that sacred Fujiyama was snow-capped. For most of us this was our first sight of snow and we drew a parallel with ourselves and the silent Mount Fuji, that long slumbered volcano, cold, desolate and alone. We had not experienced winter for many years; *taim belong kol* in New Britain could never be compared with the Japanese winter we were fated to endure.

As was the custom with Australians everywhere, we celebrated our own version of the Melbourne Cup on the first Tuesday in November, the 3rd. The day was without the usual enthusiasm, it did not seem appropriate with the temperature below freezing, snow glistening on distant mountains and no real horses to call by name.[2]

Around this time a dour looking Japanese female and several of her counterpart males arrived at the Club with bundles of different coloured yarn, which looked like silk.

'We require you to do some work for which you will be paid,' one of the men said contemptuously. After we had unwound some of this tangled 'silk' into smaller balls, the woman and some of the men demonstrated how to knit striped bags, two inches by one inch, with a fringe at the bottom. Kay asked what the bags were to be used for - they really did seem ridiculous. There was much in-drawing of breath and shuffling of feet and then one man attempted an explanation.

'Well, it is something like this and it is something to do with our religion.' Another took over and described the bags as 'card containers', which Japanese soldiers carried with them when they went into battle to keep the Americans away. To bring them good luck in general we thought! These men spoke English quite well, which didn't seem to fit in with this crazy knitting scheme; we never did understand the Japs and perhaps we never would.

We got on with this traitorous war work for which we were to receive three and a half *sen* (almost a penny) for each bag. We had become a little prudent now and scrounged everything we thought might be of use to us. This yarn was certainly classified as useful and quantities of it were carefully put out of sight. Months later, it went a long way towards the prevention of hypothermia and various complications of extreme cold that we were all destined to endure without any warm clothing.

After the completion of hundreds of these tiny bags, which was tedious work, the Japs gained the idea that we could do almost anything. One day they were having trouble moving a telephone box from one building to another and called on three of the taller girls to give them a hand. After this effort we all agreed that in the future we would appear helpless, otherwise we might be manpowered into the permanent Japanese work force.

We had long ago concluded that the Japs were inconsistent and disordered in their approach to anything practical and one day when Fuji ordered us to clean up the kitchen our ruling was confirmed.

'Me clean man no like dirt,' he stated and proceeded to throw buckets of water in all directions. Cockroaches had been preparing for winter in hung-up umbrellas and when Fuji took the umbrellas down and opened them out cockroaches scattered wildly in all directions. We were ordered to chase them with brooms and mops.

The activity became more frantic when Fuji turned his attention to where he knew, from seasons past, rats had taken up residence. He busily joined in the chase and caught one of the wretched creatures by the tail. When he held it over the open fire of the stove, we hoped it would bite him before it was incinerated, but this, unfortunately, did not happen. After the kitchen was cleaned, we tackled the bar and corners of the main rooms. This water treatment to floors and cupboards was not so bad in summer, but right now we could have been playing ice hockey. By the time Fuji and our squad had finished the place was cleaner, but the floors would probably remain wet all night.

As winter set in our food ration dwindled and we began losing weight noticeably. We knew that Fuji was cutting down our share and we complained to Tally, who was our official connection with the Foreign Office, but he was not much help. He told us of our entitlements and when we told him that these rations were followed by hordes of Fuji's friends he simply broke into laughter and it was clear to us that he was not really interested.

There was huge excitement on the 30th November when a thunderous explosion sent us scurrying onto the verandah. No alarms were sounded and no planes were heard yet a thick cloud of black smoke was billowing upwards from the harbour. That was all we could see before the Junsa hustled us inside. The reason for the sudden explosion remained a mystery until Fuji revealed, after a few days, that a tanker blew up and caught fire taking with her two other ships lying alongside. We did not know whether it was some sort of enemy espionage and we doubted if Fuji would know that either. What a bonus, three less ships for the Japs! Later, in one of his better moods, Fuji said it was a German ship that had exploded and those who had escaped were now at the Bund Hotel.[3]

'Imagine Mrs Saito being confronted with hearty eaters like the Germans and, being *allies* of the Japs, she would be forced to show them she has God in her heart!' These and other comments on

Mrs Saito's likely reactions on having to accommodate the German crew kept us entertained for some time.

The first anniversary of the bombing of Pearl Harbor, the 8th of December (Japanese time), was headlined 'America's Humiliation Day' in the *Japan Times*. We were handed a copy of this newspaper by the Junsa and given a lecture on how lucky we were to be in Japan with the kind, civilised Japanese.

'How amazing, to have bombed a country with which they were not at war and still call themselves civilised!' Their reasoning was a mystery. On this anniversary a gang of Japanese were ineffectively trying to haul Nippon's sacred flag onto the roof. This time, remembering their view of our capabilities, we all stayed inside.

Our first Christmas in captivity was approaching. Our American friend, Mrs Jones, had been given a cash donation by a representative of the Vatican to be used for American prisoners of war. With this money she was able to buy colourful paper, which the girls cut into streamers and pieces of tinsel to make adornments to help encourage a cheerful spirit with the approach of Christmas. The missionary girls, Dora Wilson and Mavis Green in particular, proved extremely talented in making decorations of flowers and little trees and even a horseshoe for luck.

On Christmas Eve we were happily taking a hand in dressing the Club for the festive season when Tally - we didn't know his real name - arrived from the Foreign Office. He looked disapprovingly at what he called this foreign idea and told us to remove *it*.

'Is that a V for Victory sign?' he asked on spotting the horseshoe. We assured him that it was not.

'Turn it upside down and you can leave it there.'

Several of us were standing on stools removing the offensive decorations and feeling sorry for the work of the artists going to such waste when a man's voice in English surprised us.

'A Happy Christmas to you all!' For a few seconds dead silence greeted his unexpected wish and the poor man stood there twirling his hat. Max Pezzalosi was a Swiss representative of the Red Cross. There were several Japanese in attendance and he informed us that his time was limited. We did manage to register a complaint with him about our lack of food and clothing and the non-existence of medical attention before the Japanese interrupted. Max proceeded to read out a Christmas message from the Australian Government and handed over boxes from the Red Cross.

'Sorry I must go now, I will try to call again soon.'

With a wave of the hand he was gone, leaving us with many suggestions and requests for the next time we would see him.

No child on Christmas morning could have been more happy and appreciative than we were when we opened our *presents* that afternoon - no one wanted to wait until tomorrow. Food was the main content of the parcels which were donated by Australia, England, South Africa and America. There were tins of biscuits, puddings, jam, syrup, cheese, pastes, tomatoes, milk, bacon and bulk packs of sugar, sweets, dried fruits, coffee and tea and the wonderful old Bully beef - one hundred tins of this.

On Christmas morning a heavy fall of snow gave us a White Christmas. There were remembrances related of sunny days and sandy beaches - and of White Cross ships that came and went - all sprinkled among carol singing and indiscriminate eating. Many of us were light-headed, having consumed large quantities of coffee, and we had just about convinced ourselves that our names would be on the list for the next exchange ship. Perhaps this was really because another winter in Japan was too terrible to contemplate. This was Christmas 1942 and it was not the end but just the beginning!

Our first winter in the northern hemisphere was something for which we were totally unprepared. Snow had fallen heavily all December and it was perishingly cold, a fitting description often expressed by residents on the New England Tableland of New South Wales when the chilling, winter winds howled in anguish in search of their destination. None of us, except Mrs Jones and Mrs Bignell, who had originally come from Scotland before settling in the islands, had ever known a White Christmas.

The snow created a pure and peaceful scene around us, but it was not the White Christmas depicted on cards at Christmas time, which to most Australians was only a dream. Those English scenes were of Christmas strangely filled with warmth, Christmas with 'sleigh bells in the snow', of people wrapped in furs and boots and muffs, of cosy fires burning in the hearth and Christmas pudding flamed with lighted brandy - a Christmas shared with the warmth of family and friends. Did that Christmas really exist? Even under the most favourable of circumstances I could only wonder what might have caused poets and song writers to become lyrical about Christmas cheer, so cold with winter snow.

The old year slipped past and wishes, both secret and not so secret, were made for the new year. On this first day of 1943 we were lined up near the frozen swimming pool and ordered to bow in the direction of the Imperial Palace. There seemed no particular reason for this homage, or the many repetitions of it that we were compelled to perform. The ritual came across as an impulsive whim on the part of our overlords, with no meaning ever explained to us.[4]

We had a day of reminiscing on January the 23rd, marking the end of our first year in captivity, and there were lots of recollections about Vunapope and of the probable fate of the missionaries. We all hoped the Americans might have made an impression by now but we really had no idea what was happening in Rabaul; all news in the *Japan Times* leaned heavily in Japan's favour. We were not even sure if our relatives knew of our fate; there had been no communication by mail allowed us in Japan. We had no way of knowing if the one letter, which we were requested to write from Vunapope, had been received, or as we began to think now - ever sent! The Japanese intended to drop these over Port Moresby but we placed little faith in this questionable delivery.[5]

In January, too, a small advertisement in the *Japan Times* caught our eye. Max, the Red Cross representative was getting married. There were no details much to our disappointment, but it prompted us to realise a conflicting perspective of this war - outside the confines of our prison peoples lives in Japan were continuing as normal.

Gert spoke to us very briefly one day as he rode past the fence, he told us that Tripoli had been evacuated by the Axis forces. Thank goodness for some good news! The *Japan Times*, with which we had been issued these last few months, had quite suddenly ceased; the tide must really be turning and we would hope for big things from now on. We were still ripening in judgement and I was ever thankful that our patience knew no bounds. With the Allied victory at Alamein last November, and now Tripoli, the tide had turned in North Africa, yet it was to be a long time before the War would end in Europe.

Before the grounds became frozen during winter we would walk about downstairs. The area around the building was enclosed and the view restricted but it did offer some privacy away from the prying eyes of old Fuji, and sometimes, from one another. An attraction down here, and the only one left to explore, was the building where the boats, belonging to the now banished Club members, were still stored. One day we found a small window not properly closed and Joyce, Whytie and I were able, not without some difficulty, to get inside.

The boats themselves were unproductive, except for some pieces of canvas, which might be useful for making summer shorts, and a few containers of no great value which were probably used in happier days for bailing out. The canvas-covered guard house had been badly shredded by the wind but it too gave us some useful cloth. While the three of us were rummaging around inside and under the boats Kay appeared and retrieved the small electric cooker which we had left alone. We didn't have Kay's knowledge of electricity! Kay rigged the little stove up in the shower room and it gave wonderful service when we were able to acquire rice and vegetables. Mysteriously, the lights failed a few times but were soon put right by our useful electrician.

As winter dragged on our food ration decreased even further and we were always hungry and losing more weight. When Tally paid another visit he condescended to listen to our grievances and then went on to tell us, over again, that rations consisted of a bowl of rice three times a day, vegetables, fish, and two loaves of bread (when it was obtainable). It was a forgone conclusion that he did not believe our stories, or did not want to, especially after his interviews with Fuji. That old devil always gave us a good meal when officials arrived which gave no support to our case. Many times we saw Fuji's friends from the new barge building yards, in front of the Club, lining up at the kitchen; the Junsa, too, was seen to join the food queue.

A frequent visitor to the Club was Mori whom Fuji said was the head buyer of food for all the camps. Added to the local hangers on Mori and other officials received oddments of tools and items of hardware from the workers on the waterfront. We called this exchange bribery!

When the warmer weather came we struggled to dig a vegetable plot inside the fence and planted seeds from vegetables scrounged by various means. When our skimpy crop reached full growth, many products of the yield, mainly pumpkins, disappeared before we could lay our hands on them, which was very disheartening, but we persevered nevertheless.

On the Emperor's birthday, the 29th April, we were once again lined up to bow in the direction of the palace. Hundreds of planes flew over Tokyo and as we were watching them old Fuji came out and bared his dirty teeth in something resembling a grin.

'Plenty more have got,' he said, just in case we might think this was the entire strength of Dai Nippon's Air Force!

Soon after this aerial display Max (the Red Cross representative we had met at Christmas) arrived with a crowd of coolies. We found it strange and very disappointing that we were not permitted to contact him, and it seemed that he was not permitted to contact us either. We watched with interest and some misgivings, as the workmen climbed up through the manhole in the boat-house and dragged out furniture, cutlery and linen and last, but not least, a gramophone. We contemplated at one stage unlocking the secrets beyond the manhole, but decided that there would be only exposed wires, rats, and probably snakes up there. And now, to find out we had missed this booty was really quite shattering, especially the gramophone and the linen.

A few days after the visitors with the furniture van had left, important Army and Navy officials began inspecting the downstairs rooms. They prowled around and made sweeping gestures indicating large areas around the building. All this activity puzzled us and, for once, no one was able to come forward with any clue - one or two of us would usually have something to offer. Old Fuji, too, was strangely quiet and very busy as he prepared endless meals for these distinguished visitors. He made a real Japanese delicacy, *Sashimi*, for them. It was actually raw fish prepared with vinegar and sliced in different ways to bring out the flavour and not something our palates could easily accept. Fuji served it with soy sauce and freshly grated horseradish, but not to us and I must say that although we were very hungry we would have been reluctant to taste this delight.

When the Army and Navy personnel departed Fuji immediately started hauling plates and cutlery from the Club storage and set us on a washing-up campaign. Our mounting curiosity and obvious excitement must have finally got through to Fuji.

'Seventy big Naval men, same as you (meaning prisoners) coming live downstairs,' he blurted out, unable to contain himself any longer.

Excitement mounted the next day when the Junsa ordered that we were not to go near the windows overlooking the entrance gate, we were to stay out of the kitchen where a clear view from the windows could be had. The usual thing happened, the one-track mind of the Japs forgot the bathroom windows downstairs that were immediately under the kitchen windows!

We maintained dead silence upstairs as we sat around pretending to read, while listening for every sound. Two of the girls went below to take the first watch. We had no idea when the *big men* were expected. Obviously Fuji hadn't any information either as he liked to be first with the news on these occasions. Nearly an hour had gone by when Whytie appeared from below.

'Only one man has arrived,' she announced, 'and you'll never guess who it is.'

'Flying Officer Geoffrey Lempriere!' Whytie exclaimed.

Geoffrey Lempriere was one of the eight who had been living downstairs when we first arrived at the Club, he was the RAAF Intelligence Officer from the Rabaul Squadron.[6] No one else arrived and we never did find out what happened to the rest of the *big men*; if they ever existed except in the imagination of the Japs.

No one knew who started calling our new neighbour Ducky. When we told Geoffrey of his nickname he agreed that it was anonymous enough not to attract the notice of the Junsa or Fuji. Our communications followed the same pattern as before when the men were down below last year.

Ducky wrote items of news from the *Times* and wrapped them in sanitary paper or soap paper. These messages came flying over the verandah wall when the opportunity arose, mostly when he was out on PT in the earlier days. However, as time went by, the Junsa became bored having only one prisoner to watch and his absences increased. We posted look-outs for his return and were able to have many interesting conversations, which passed the time and relieved the dreariness, especially for Ducky.

News about the exchange ships which were operating regularly could still fill our minds with hope and cause a flurry of inspection of wardrobes. Ducky told us that there were many requests in the *Japan Times* for supplies of soya bean curd, pickles and similar delicacies to be sent to the Japanese people languishing in Allied internment camps. He was supplied with a daily issue of the *Japan Times* and was instructed to comment about the likely results of the war and Japan's role in the conflict - 'without fear of repercussion'. A different official quizzed him from time to time and when this took place under our verandah we listened carefully to these interrogations.

When the spring rains came Ducky underwent a period of what was virtually solitary confinement. During this time the rain fell in torrents without a break for several days and his guard, who was no doubt feeling almost a prisoner himself, locked the doors and windows and disappeared for long periods. The continual dampness from the wet weather caused Ducky to suffer bouts of malaria, but worst of all he told us later was the lack of communication. He was amazed that the Japs had brought him here at all. They could have got 'his views' just as easily at Ofuna camp where his companions were at present and from whence he had come.

When the sun shone again the news bulletins continued. We were not to put in writing anything he told us about the Naval Interrogation camp at Ofuna, which was south of Tokyo and not all that far from here. Allied prisoners, from aircraft carriers, PBYs

(Catalinas) and submarines, were grilled and cruelly beaten at this camp, "but the other prisoners were not able, at this date, to exchange details as they were kept separated and cross examined individually".

Ducky had been downstairs for several weeks. He told us one day that he thought the guard was suspicious about his communication with us. Shortly after this, when let out for exercise, he saw the Jap conceal himself under our verandah instead of going off to talk to someone on the premises as was usual. Of course there was no conversation that day and we were more careful about being conspicuous for a while. We had become, over a period, accustomed to the inconsistencies of the Japs and were not too surprised when, a few days later, Ducky's guard went out fishing with Kimura. He had ordered our Junsa to keep an eye on Ducky downstairs. However, our guard (the *Go* addict) became involved in a game and forgot all about Ducky. Taking advantage of this good fortune we took turns and talked for nearly two hours while writing messages and absorbing information to take to Australia if we were exchanged.

A few days later there was a loud *Sayonara* from below and soon afterwards Ducky and his guard left. We hoped that he would soon have the company of his friends and live to see the Allies arrive.

More depressed than usual after Ducky's departure, a few of us took advantage of our *Go* guard once more and escaped downstairs, climbed down the ladder and swam in the filthy, oily waters of Tokyo Bay. An awful way to break the monotony!

Old Fuji, always demanding to be addressed as Fujita San, was a great thorn in our side, one of the reasons being that he understood Europeans more than any other Japanese who had been in contact with us. We felt as if he could read our minds. In these early days at the Club, before he became constantly *bubbly* (explosive), he told us he was once chief cook on a ship. It seemed this was an English or Australian vessel as Fuji had visited Australia many times. We often discussed his continually venomous attitude towards us and wondered if he had received similar treatment from some of his former superiors. Fuji had very keen hearing and we were certain he knew what we were saying when we whispered to each other.

As time went by there seemed to be no doubt that Fujita San's role was to spy on us. He was invaluable to the guards and others as an interpreter. Any new guard, who was reasonably affable towards us at the beginning, would change his attitude after morning tea sessions with Fuji and look on us with far more jaundiced eye. Often, when we were working in the kitchen, Fuji would bang his cleaver on the wooden table and make threatening remarks towards us.

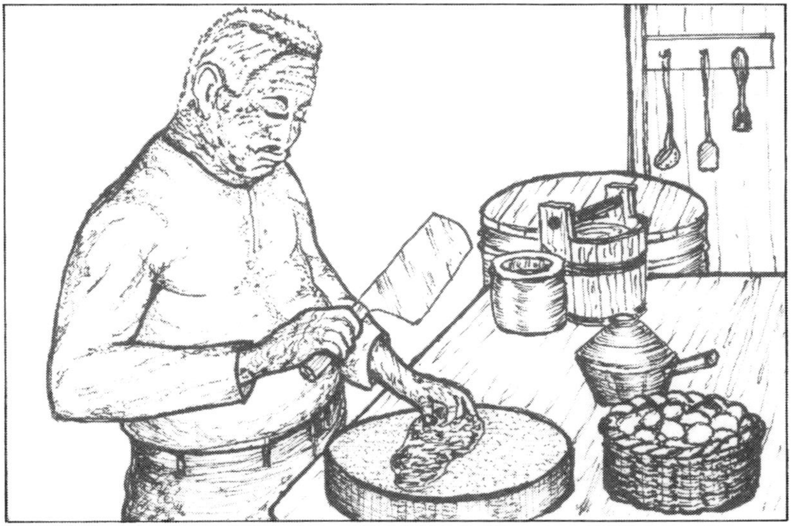

Fuji banging his cleaver

'More better Junsa beat you, more better you die. Japanese soldier like die, no like come back.'

During these episodes we were petrified with fright. Our Japanese interpreting book told us that Fuji meant fire and I thought his mother had named him appropriately.

The anniversary of Emperor Meiji's birthday, August 30th, was always a day of great celebration for Japan; on this holiday aquatic sports took place in the vicinity of the Yokohama Yacht Club. Emperor Meiji, the great-grandfather of the present Son of Heaven, Hirohito, was highly esteemed and was the last feudal Emperor of Japan. The new constitution of Japan was based on the philosophy of the Meiji period. We were all full of curiosity about the forthcoming celebrations and looking forward to seeing them, if only through the peep-holes on the verandah.

The next few days however brought a sequence of events that drove everything else out of our minds. The Undertaker, the man who had taken charge of us when we arrived last year, came to see us.

'Be ready to move from here in a few days.'

Excitement mounted and reached a peak of almost hysterical level, when later that day a White Cross ship came into the harbour - we had not seen one since the spring. Officials had neither confirmed nor denied that we might be exchanged and when we tried to pump old Fuji for information he would yell at us and become even more *bubbly* than his usual cantankerous self.

'No my business, my business cook business.'

From the time of the ship's arrival onward our receptive minds gobbled up everything that sounded even remotely feasible.

'You know that man who was here yesterday,' remarked Mrs Jones, referring to the Undertaker, 'well, I've been trying to think where I have seen him before - he was right there when I came off the ship from the Aleutians.' Mrs Jones seldom held out any hope of being exchanged, yet her almost casual comment strengthened our theory that the Undertaker was in charge of shipping.

In between pulling bags and cases from under our *tatami* (sleeping mats), bringing out the special dress we had shut away and salvaging any make-up still useable, we took turns in keeping watch below. We hoped to be able to contact Gert who might have some information about exchange arrangements. When Gert did appear in the distance, in the late afternoon, he waved and indicated that he was unable to get near the low fence that separated the vacant land and barge buildings further away. This was the last time we ever saw him.

After a sleepless night and a scanty bowl of rice the Junsa ordered us downstairs. Silence, that comes with anticipation - not wanting anything to go wrong - took the place of excitement now when the *Black Maria* arrived and the Junsa shepherded us aboard.

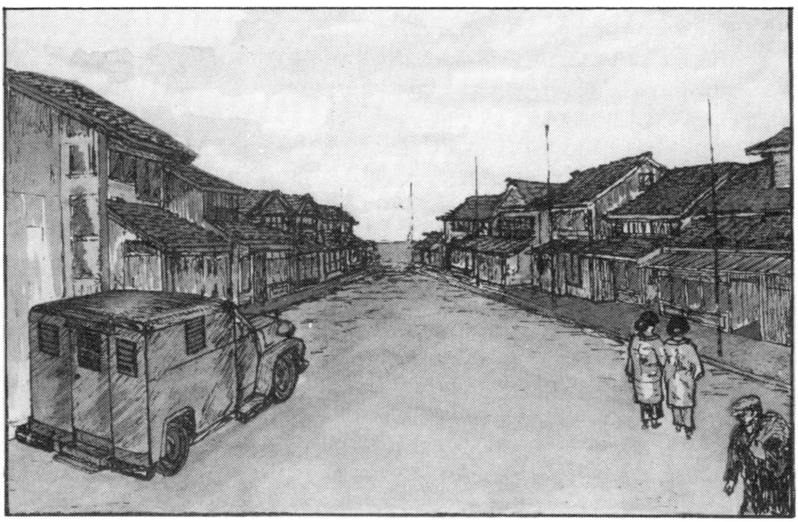

No sight of the Harbour

We were somewhat subdued as we travelled through suburban streets, with no sight of the harbour. It wasn't long before the vehicle came to a halt inside the courtyard of a large building and our hopes were still with us when the guard opened the door. This was probably a transit centre and we would join other people here. We gathered our luggage and the Junsa ordered us upstairs.

This important looking place was actually the headquarters of the Kanagawa Prefecture. We were assembled in a very large room which was obviously used for teaching purposes; it was packed with solid looking desks and benches and was the first floor of this three-storey building. It was to be our quarters; we were going nowhere!

As this was the only room allotted to us we set-to and moved the desks and benches against the walls and placed tables in convenient places for sleeping. Later tatami were brought in and placed on the tables. This heavy manual work helped in a small way to take our minds off the morning's terrible disappointment, though none of us had really given up entirely. Trivial as it would have seemed under ordinary circumstances the move to these premises, and the surroundings, provided a welcome diversion for our troubled minds.

This large room, furnished like a modern Western lecture room, did not prepare us for the shock on sighting the amenities on the floor below. Here the toilets were slits in the floor in an area only partly partitioned off, and at one end, in view of all comers, were rows of urinals. These toilets were used by both sexes and were the only ones in the building, which had not been built for a high degree of occupancy. There were no showers or baths here. On emerging from the 'little room' one was frequently greeted with a polite *konnichi wa* (good-day) from a man at the urinal section. Two of us usually visited these regions together - one keeping guard as it were.

One day I was on guard duty and was sitting on the stairs when a man came along and gave me an inquiring look. I did not know enough Japanese at this stage to tell him that there was someone in there so I just waved my hand in the general direction and suggested he'd better try the others as they were all free. When he came out he paused on the stairs, spoke, but did not wait for a reply.

'Australian?' he quietly questioned.

Interesting as the sea could sometimes be at the Club we soon discovered there were far more diverse interests here. It was relaxing for us too, the Junsa had more company and often left us to our own devices. We were not supposed *to see* or *to be seen*, but as usual, we found plenty of opportunities to find loopholes in this rule.

The street below was lined with beautiful trees and the leaves were already touched with the bronze and gold of early autumn. The fan-like, divided leaf of the *Iche* was a lovely sight among the ornamental pines and spruce. The Japanese seem to specialise in trees and at the Yacht Club we saw them transplant fully grown trees on the waterfront without any loss at all. Perhaps the Japanese deserved the title attributed to them as the world's best gardeners.

Large pillars inside this huge room partly obscured the windows, but they came in very handy as a hiding place, and from here we had excellent vision across the way. The buildings opposite were comfortable looking flats with an assortment of seemingly interesting tenants of various nationalities. They appeared to be leading normal lives and because of this we were intrigued.

Soon after taking up a viewing position, not long after our arrival, I observed identical twins waddle into the room opening onto the balcony opposite. These tubby, middle aged men, who looked to be Italians, seated themselves at a table and a Japanese girl in a white *kimono* proceeded to fill their glasses from a wine jar. Later she produced a tray laden with food. A few of the other girls joined me and we watched with fascination as the mountainous pile was demolished, interspersed with emptying and filling of wine glasses. Our envy and nostalgia reached its peak when a little later the maid placed what resembled a pineapple in front of these two. We began to wonder about our own food and what arrangements had been made in that regard. Our query was soon answered when almost like an apparition old Fuji appeared with our meal in containers.

A pack of playing cards one of the girls brought from the Club got a face-lift one day when Kay found a well of red ink in one of the desks. We played bridge between intervals of street watching and waiting for Fuji to arrive with our daily rice ration. Although there were no cooking facilities here we were not as hungry as we were at the Club. Fuji, as we guessed, would not and did not have the nerve to cut our rice down to below subsistence level under the eyes of these guards he'd not been able to 'work on'.

Fuji always came on a bicycle, with our food perched in front of him, and it was our great worry that he might have an accident. The worst did happen one day and the old boy arrived almost incoherent with a sad tale that he'd been 'knocked off bike'. Fuji rose a little in our estimation when we found most of the food intact, though some was mixed with gravel from the streets of Yokohama.

One morning, when the Junsa was not around, Joyce and I took a stroll down the passage and came to an open room lined with shelves on which there were bundles of clothing, suitcases, umbrellas and other odds and ends, giving it the appearance of a second-hand shop. At first we thought that these goods had probably been taken from internees, but found that they were all of Japanese origin and this room was really the lost property office. Perhaps there was something honest about the Japanese after all.

That afternoon the sound of singing in the street brought us all rushing to the windows of our quarters. The Junsa was absent and it was wonderful to hear the lively music of a European marching song. We felt a spark of remorse on finding out later that we had enjoyed the singing of Germans on their way to the German Club.

Another day when we were downstairs doing some washing in the basins, a bloated middle-aged man with a pasty face came stumbling down the stairs from the floor above. He was under guard and looked straight ahead appearing totally unaware that we were giving him all our attention. We watched when he crossed the courtyard and was taken into another wing of the building. He belonged to the Nordic race and we decided he must be a political prisoner. We saw him again, twice, after this and each time he behaved as though he were a zombie. On the last occasion he walked away from his guards and came towards us. We were about to speak but he did not so much as glance in our direction; he spat into the nearest basin and returned to his guards. It wasn't often we were thwarted in an effort to have our curiosity satisfied, but we were never able to find out anything about this stranger.

In another part of the building there were rooms with bars on the windows. This place was near the toilets and middle aged Japanese women with keys dangling from their waists were frequently seen going in and out of the rooms. One day when one of these attendants came close to us we asked her who was in there.

'Prisoners,' was the laconic reply.

'Like us?'

'No, bad girls.'

We never did see these 'bad girls', but they had our sympathy. There is nothing like being confined against one's will to stir up a fellow-feeling. If they were prisoners of their own destiny, perhaps it was not a destiny willingly chosen in these trying times.

The two-storey apartment next to us was the residence of the Chief of Police of the Foreign Office. Two families were apparently living there and numerous children played in the courtyard. A nurse in a white uniform was always in attendance and she often brought a baby down in a pram, or push-cart, for an airing. The Chief and his second in command - both in shirt sleeves - paid us an informal visit one day. They were quite pleasant, but dispassionate, as they took a quick look around and left. On the way out the Chief spotted a pot of flourishing mint and the half-grown pumpkin one of the girls had rescued from under the heels of the workman outside the Club. For some reason this homely sight seemed to amuse them and they laughed heartily as they went down the stairs.

As well as occupants of the buildings coming under our scrutiny, there were many more people to interest us passing in the street below.

In contrast to the women looking like moving flower stems in *kimonos*, there were others in a strange version of trousers. These pants were the Government's idea of appropriate wartime attire for women, something of a uniform, but actually traditionally worn in the fields by peasant women. This atrocity, known as a *mompei*, started off as a skirt pleated around a waistband, then it divided above the knees and gathered again a few inches above the ankle forming balloon type trousers, which, to some extent, concealed the bandy legs of the wearer.

To protect them from sun and rain the Japanese carried umbrellas of many colours which were made with oiled paper stretched over a frame of fine bamboo ribs. In the very early woodblock prints by Japanese artists the umbrella, or *karakasa* as it is called, gave a token of grace and beauty to the traditional scene. Not so though, the most incongruous scene to behold in the street below. Riding along on their bicycles uniformed police, under gaily coloured umbrellas, carried their belongings in bundles wrapped in gaily coloured material. Regardless of uniform or station we observed that everyone transported possessions in this way. We were reminded of the very first Japanese we had seen at Vunapope wrapping their loot from the fruit trees in the bright squares of cloth and we learned in time that these cloth bundles have a special Japanese name, the *furoshiki*.

The coolies in their large hats and *happi* coats, again gaily coloured, were everywhere. They could be seen running between the shafts of rickshaws or pulling wooden carts filled with everything from household furniture to fowls, children sitting among stacks of clothing or just plain rubbish. The coolie's *happi* coat might look, spell and sound like a 'happy' coat, but this workman's garb is perhaps the direct opposite to the implied meaning of our English word. The strangest sight of all to us were Japanese men wearing only a loincloth, the *fundoshi*, who were also carrying umbrellas - some, oddly enough, were wearing Wellington boots! The workman at the building yards near the Club were often seen in this garb in the summer and we formed the conclusion, after seeing them in the street, that it was a traditional type of garment, as also seemed to be the khaki attire, buttoned to the neck, worn by most workers in winter. The whole cosmopolitan street scene was most unusual and gave us as much entertainment as any stage show.

One of the most amusing of the street pantomimes was what we called The Air Raid Practice. Masses of little women converged on the street below one warm afternoon. They were all dressed alike in the hideous *mompei* and had handkerchiefs tied around their heads; they clip-clopped around looking like a busy group in fancy dress. The sound that echoed from the street as their wooden *geta* beat a tattoo was rather like that of trotting ponies. This active little group seized hoses, and water squirted everywhere; the rest of the squad hit the pavement wildly with their mats. When a number of these little ladies tripped over the hoses, ending with their bottoms in the air, we got our first laugh for a long time as they fought to extricate themselves. Half drowned and with their trousers ballooning out from the waist they looked like beer barrels rolling around the street. After this display another group arrived and let off a *smoke bomb*; this was the signal for the First Aid to get into action. These donned masks, shut windows and then collected the 'wounded' and carted them into 'our' courtyard where the fracture cases were splinted and bandaged. With the arrival of the ambulance the injured, who were not too competently handled, were bundled inside.

The guards told us later that the commotion we had *heard* in the street below was practice in preparation for possible attacks on harmless civilians by none other than the barbarous Americans!

'You will go back to the *boato* Club today,' the Junsa told us. And so our 'vacation' came to an end.

Two weeks had passed and our awareness of the neighbourhood and its many nationalities had been both engrossing and enlightening. This was not bad really for a group who was supposed *not to see* and *not be seen by* the passers by. Now we were to return to the *boato* Club. In a way it had been a kind of vacation; the guards were rarely present and best of all was the absence of surveillance by that old devil Fujita San. There had been little talk about exchange ships during this period. After our initial disappointment it would have been tempting fate to have even thought about this mind disturbing subject.

'Well there doesn't seem to be any doubt about our

destination this time,' Joyce said. 'Do you think we'll have to move all this furniture back into place before we go?'

There was no doubt about that either and after more than an hour of dragging and heaving, the room reverted to lecture room orderliness once again. Nineteen dispassionate workers went below for a final clean-up before another ride in the *Black Maria*.

On arrival at the Club it was evident that there had been considerable activity during our absence. Small low buildings lined the waterfront and the vacant land where Gert and his companion rode their horses was alive with more barge construction works, where men, women and children seemed to be eagerly working.

'This place will make a good target for the boys when they come over,' one of the girls said as we dropped out of *Maria*.

'Well if that happens none of us will be around to clear up the debris.'

Visitors had viewed the celebrations of the Emperor's birthday from the Club verandah. The wooden fence up there had been removed and roughly put back and there were more peep-holes than previously. The fence right around the Club had been removed altogether and there were no signs of the gardens we had battled with all summer. Walking outdoors was forbidden now and when we observed the exchange ship - or was it another one - at anchor in the harbour we adopted a low profile.

Kimura, the former Club steward had been around in one capacity or another from the time we arrived at the Club. He had to date been able to skirt being called up to do his bit for Emperor and country, but was at last summoned to Tokyo to join-up. This was very pleasing news as far as we were concerned; his absence made one less Jap around to spy on us. Kimura had always presented a particular untrusting presence and we were pleased to be rid of him.

Sometimes, in Fuji's rare absence, Mori would come over from the other camp where the 'rich men' were interned. Where this camp was we did not know. He would prowl around in the kitchen and finally come storming out in a rage (perhaps assumed) and tell us "Fuji is a thief and a blackguard". He would report him to the Foreign Office, and we would get more food. When Fuji returned we told him of Mori's visit, and of his comments.

Fuji's reactions never ceased to amaze us. He made no denial about the accusations and immediately handed out presents of fat, tea, rice cakes and salt to us. The rice cakes had rather a greyish tinge, but things like that didn't worry us too much now. A few weeks later we caught Fuji giving one of his *piecees* (relatives) about twenty pounds of uncooked rice. Following this roguery we got almost our full quota of food for a week!

Another winter was beginning and we could not see how we would get through it. We were without even the basic clothing now for protection against the bitter cold soon to be upon us. Strangely, under these circumstances inventive minds started working and after much trial and error the Goshu (Australian) Weaving Company was launched. The raw materials for this venture were the balls of 'silk', left overs from the soldiers' card bags, made last year - those that were intended to keep the Japanese soldiers from harm when in combat with the Americans. The 'wool' comprised the rolls of cotton wool brought with us from Rabaul, a gift from the nuns at Vunapope, and even fragments from *Priscilla*; these sanitary pads were no longer needed as malnutrition advanced. Razor blades completed the equipment necessary to set up the factory.

The yarn was unravelled to whatever ply was needed and wisps of cotton wool were rolled into this using a shaven leg. This was a tedious undertaking but with so many legs available the balls of wool increased surprisingly fast. The workers proved adept and became competitive, and there was talk of offering the patent to Paton and Baldwin after the war! Much patience was needed in the knitting of this yarn with our bamboo needles but, when the composed knitters had overcome initial difficulties, amazingly attractive, warm jerseys were the result.[7]

December was upon us and it was time to think about Christmas cheer though we had no real desire to celebrate Christmas. As the day drew near a few of the girls, again this year under the supervision of Dora and Mavis, cheered us with their talents for making something really appealing out of virtually nothing. Dora and Mavis were wizards with paper and crayons and set the girls to work with the ever useful razor blade, cutting out artistic designs on coloured paper to make place mats. They created graceful waterlilies out of the same material; the mirror in the shower room was unscrewed and these works of art when placed on the table looked beautiful reflected in the glass. For Mrs Jones the girls made a fir tree and covered the branches with white wool, and for the rest of us they created miniature wattle trees, the branches laden with little yellow balls.

On Christmas Day we had a wonderful surprise - the Undertaker arrived from the Foreign Office with boxes of marvellous gifts from the Red Cross. We honoured the hallowed day as usual, but could not hide a touch of anxiety. That night we were unable to sleep with acute indigestion after feasting on bully beef, raisins and other delicacies and drinking innumerable cups of black coffee. In the parcels as well were cakes of soap and other necessary items which had been denied us, but, of course, our main pleasure was gleaned from the edible provisions.

In spite of all attempts to keep our spirits high, the downward path had accelerated over these last months. Our general health and morale reached a very low ebb and there was more strife in store for us when a sour, middle aged woman joined Fuji in the kitchen. We decided she had been sent to spy on us and perhaps Fuji as well. Her name was Moricame and as time went by it was obvious that Fuji was afraid of her; he referred to her as that crazy no-good woman.

As far as we were concerned it wasn't long before there was worse to come. Up to now our various guards, generally, had been indifferent and bored, frequently giving the impression that guarding a bunch of females lowered their status. All this changed with the arrival of Komatz and Basher, who embarked upon their guard-duty with zeal. We never knew the latter's real name but he sure did earn the title we gave him. These two had been recently discharged from the Army and saw their assignment as necessary justification to create havoc for us. Komatz was obviously very sick; our diagnosis of his condition was an advanced stage of Tuberculosis and that he was, also, quite mad. The woman Moricame seemed to be in league with these two and old Fuji became an outsider; over this period we almost felt some sympathy for him.

Ever since we had come to the Club one of our chores was to take the guard's meal, on a tray, to his room. He would usually just grunt or ignore us entirely when we put his food on the low table.

The first morning after the arrival of these new overlords I was doing kitchen chores. I took the rice and pickle breakfast to Komatz in the usual manner and found that my performance did not meet with his approval. In spite of his illness, he jumped to his feet like an agile animal and proceeded to give me a demonstration on how to present, correctly, his food. The ritual was to bow very low and say in Japanese 'Deign to accept this honourable food', and while still bowing withdraw from the room by taking steps backwards to the door. After breakfast Moricame took me aside and introduced me to some more of the niceties of Japanese etiquette when removing the tray from his lordship's presence.

Basher was just as vicious in his attitude towards us but he had one diversion - he was in love - or at least appeared to be and disappeared for long intervals with his girlfriend. This set-up suited us, especially at night, as he didn't spend time darting in and out, as did Komatz, to make sure we were kept out of bed. We referred to Basher's girl as Sweetie Pie and thought that old Fuji was not aware of this pseudonym; of course we were wrong as usual. Fuji knew us too well now to be taken in by most of our attempts at cover-up. Although Fuji was terrified of both Basher and Komatz he was rather prudish and did not approve of our frivolous remarks about the pair.

One day when Joyce and I were talking about them Fuji gave us a very dirty look.

'She no sweetheart she auntie, you savvy, sister belong poppa.' We savvied and made a note to be a bit more cautious in the future.

Not long after this Joyce took Basher his supper one evening when Sweetie Pie was visiting. Liklik and I were wondering whether we dare go to bed when Joyce finally appeared after cleaning up the kitchen.

'What's going on in there?' I nodded towards Basher's room.

'Well, everything seemed quiet, when I left him he was busy with a hot savoury dish,' she said innocently and was quite annoyed when we burst out laughing.

'It doesn't take much to amuse you these days,' came her injured response.

After two years with the Japanese we could still be surprised when, for no perceivable reason their minds would suddenly switch to another track. One night, when we were lined up for *Tenko* by Komatz anticipating, as usual, his ranting and raving, he simply looked us over quietly and lunged toward us tapping four of the girls on the shoulder. He beckoned them forward, and we held our breath. Plainly enjoying the suspense he, slowly, but very consciously, began to praise them for good works and behaviour. After this it took a long time for those four to live down the reputation of KPs - Komatz' Pets.

As time went on Basher and Komatz caused intense anxiety among us, and sometimes outright terror not knowing what to expect. They made an awful fuss about their food and we wondered if old Fuji would end up having a breakdown and commit *harakiri*, he had become very subdued and yielding, even in *our* presence. The aggressive female Moricame had become wary of these two bullies as well and was now servile in their company. Komatz used to cough up blood and spit all over the place, including the kitchen. On these occasions Fuji stood rigidly at attention and bellowed at us to clean up the mess. If Komatz remained present, in spite of what we considered his almost terminal condition, he would spring madly into the air and slap our faces or strike us with the butt of his rifle. These exertions brought on further coughing fits. He went totally berserk when in these frenzied states and would cease, only, when utterly exhausted.

Tenko, these days and nights, became a full dress affair. The procedure adopted by both Basher and Komatz, when we were lined up for the ritual, was always the same; cap and gloves would be removed slowly and the ever gleaming sword brandished, while looking us over. Komatz would walk tediously up to the recipient of his scrutiny and slap her face. In the case of the taller girls he would stand on his toes, all the while screaming *baka* (fool). After this display he was always on the verge of collapse. On recovering his breath he sheathed his sword, which brought audible sighs of relief, yet, neither of them would be finished with us so lightly. Komatz aspired to inflame us with Japanese language lessons, whereas Basher gave testimony to his name.

'The cherry blossoms bloom in the spring and are very pretty.' We had to repeat over and over for Komatz on these wretchedly cold nights in winter. He did not think talking about flowers in the springtime inappropriate under the circumstances.[8]

'The third month in Japan is *taihen astui* (very hot).' Totally untrue I wanted to yell. We certainly didn't appreciate standing there slowly freezing and being told what to expect in a few months. If Komatz could have his wish granted we would not be alive then anyway. After about half an hour of this futile session, when our inquisitor began to wilt, we were dismissed, but not allowed to retire. We were so stiff with cold we could hardly move!

In the past under more rational guards, *Tenko* would finish and, after much bowing and saying *O-yasumi nasai* (please rest well), we were then dismissed and free to go our way. Basher and Komatz put an end to this routine. We now had to sit around freezing after being dismissed, while they huddled around the warmth of the *hibachi* and darted out at intervals to make sure that we were not going to bed. This went on for however long it suited them or until they retired. The first night of the language lessons Komatz did not reappear and we finally decided to go to bed, somewhat hopefully wondering if he might not have gone to his Shinto heaven!

One night after a session when Kay had been the recipient of the face slapping, Basher became more unhinged than usual and while unsheathing his sword walked back a few paces from the centre of the line-up. Yelling like the maniac he was he made a sudden lunge towards Joyce. Had Joyce not taken a very quick step to the side, she would most certainly have been run through.

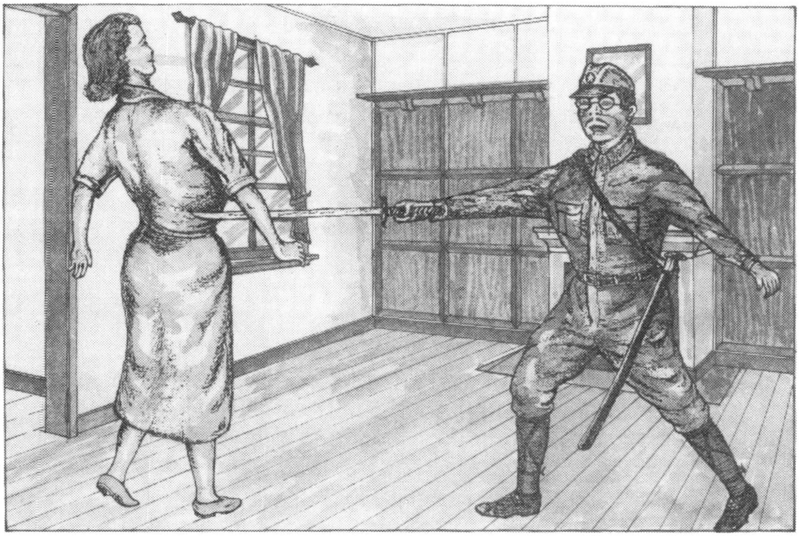

Joyce taking a very quick step to the side

The next morning when I was cleaning Komatz' room I picked up the bucket just as he appeared looking ready for trouble. He let out an animal like scream while making a spring in my direction and in a flash a ju-jitzu hold laid me flat on the floor. The contact with the floor stunned me for a few seconds and the next thing I heard was the commotion at the door as I saw Komatz attempting to rise from the floor beside me. The girls had witnessed his fall, during the execution of my humiliation, and this had surely caused him to lose face. He was now so exhausted and wheezy that he was unable to speak. Fortunately he didn't appear again that day though I got little sympathy from my friends over the episode.

'You should have tried harder and put up more resistance and you might have killed him, or at least injured the lunatic and we could have rushed in and rendered first aid,' Liklik uttered enthusiastically.

'And of course, Komatz being a Jap and incapable of showing gratitude for such a favour would have to do the 'honourable thing' and all our problems would be solved,' added Whytie.

'Very funny,' I said. 'You can have the honour of sending him to his Shinto heaven next time!'

Winter crawled slowly towards spring and the terrible monotony of being confined upstairs contributed immensely to our misery. The boat buildings along the waterfront progressed almost up to the Club since the removal of the fence around it, and this was the reason given for our confinement.

We did get downstairs occasionally when we emptied the garbage pail, which we were grateful to do since we salvaged a few odds and ends from it, the best items being orange peelings which did make a difference to the tasteless rice. When Fuji needed fuel for the stove two of us would be sent below also, with buckets, to collect coal from a small storage-house. We noticed on one of these 'outings' that Fuji had been throwing the ashes out of the kitchen window and the heap was creeping up the wall almost to the bathroom windows. It appeared Komatz had noticed it too.

One bitterly cold, windy afternoon found Komatz in one of his particularly venomous moods and we were ordered to move the ash pile away from the building. Much as we all wanted to go outside the thought of being caught up in swirls of ash and soot in the biting wind was daunting to say the least.

'What about telling Komatz that this is going to be very bad for his chest?' suggested Whytie, who must have been feeling inadvertently brave.

'Let's get on with it and hope it finishes him off,' I said, thinking this was a better idea.

Komatz had decided that we were to empty the ash over the sea wall and fussed about giving orders in his not very strong voice, until a coughing fit stopped him. Kay took over and indicated to us to take up the wooden pails stacked against the wall.

'This is going to take all afternoon girls, we'd better get started.'

The wind was strong and swirled and changed continually and we were covered in ash from head to foot. We looked like Eskimos in a snow storm without fur coats for protection. Komatz stood stolidly nearby scorning the slight shelter of the wall like a true soldier of Nippon - he would never abandon his post and lose face. Some of us almost felt sorry for the poor wretch in his weakened state. Hours later the work was finished and so were we. The wind had changed once again and there was almost as much grey powder on the ground by the sea wall as there was floating on the sea surface.

Upstairs at last, we faced another challenge, the cold shower. Some of the girls were for jumping under the icy water as they were and peeling clothes off as they soaked themselves. Others said it would be better to cover up the windows and shut out the sight of the snow. Whichever way it was done it needed a lot of will-power, which we managed to find somehow; it took us a while but in the end we were all washed. We declined the advice of Mrs Jones, to bathe like the Eskimos do during the freezing winter. Mrs Jones quietly told us how they prepared their bodies with seal oil, then sat in front of a smouldering fire, in a tightly closed room, until almost overcome with heat. She continued the story of how, when on the point of unconsciousness, they stumbled out into sub-zero weather and rubbed themselves vigorously with snow, completing the cleansing by beating each other with branches from the fir trees.

'And it didn't make them smell one bit sweeter,' she added in her slow American accent. She hastened to add that she had never seen Eskimo women take a bath in this way!

Mrs Jones had lived in Alaska for twenty years and often related wonderful tales of Eskimos and Indians, of whales and seals and the fur trade. She had trained as a nurse and as a teacher and was a very capable woman; her stories helped pass many weary hours. The loss of her husband was a shocking experience yet she hid in her heart her bitter thoughts, but would never forget his brutal and unnecessary murder by the Japs.

Our physical condition had greatly deteriorated as winter was coming to an end, yet spring, which we hoped might improve the food supply, was still a few months ahead. The sighting of maps in the Japanese newspapers gave us a clear indication that the Allies were gaining ground in Europe and Africa; amidst all our misery this gave a glimmer of renewed hope.

For some time now, there had been hints by Fuji and the Foreign Office officials that we would be moved to the country and that we would not like it there. The Japs, when trying to impart bits of information, generally got bogged down in the effort to express themselves and we heard this news in *spurts and jerks*, as one of the girls put it. A worrying announcement was: "No water there". We got the idea that these prophets of doom did not want to leave their homes in the city and it was *they* who would not like it there.

The general opinion among us was that, although this Club house was comfortable enough, if the food problem became worse we could not survive another winter here, and it was quite probable that there would be more food in the country. Another bit of information, which came from Mori who seemed to be residing at the Club now, was that people were leaving the cities for country areas.

'The Army wants this building,' he added.

We waited patiently without becoming too enthusiastic about a move that might or might not find us better off. And by now, we no longer expected to be exchanged on White Cross ships!

Meanwhile an official from the Foreign Office arrived one day with huge stacks of newspaper. The bundles were stacked in the Club's public room and the pile reached more than half-way to the ceiling. The paper on closer inspection was found to be cut into small squares. Many not yet cut up were printed in English, but the most astonishing thing was the date. They had been printed during the last war in 1916 and 1917!

The purpose of this *presento* was envelope production, another war effort. We were given small brushes and tins of powder to which water was to be added and cooked until thick. This was the glue. As this work was official Fuji was forced to allow us to cook the glue on his stove. Each day the glue making went on for longer periods than necessary depending on the odds and ends of rice and vegetables we were able to scrounge, and illicitly cook.

Our homemade glue looked rather revolting, but one by one we were tempted to taste it and the verdict was "like a nasty, sticky porridge". Before settling down to a morning's envelope-making a good portion of glue was secretly spooned into a tin and taken downstairs to the bathroom. In the process of our envelope work it was necessary to get up at intervals and walk about clapping hands to get the circulation going, and during these periods we would disappear downstairs for a snack of glue. The envelope industry progressed very slowly!

Maisie had long suffered from recurrent bouts of malaria and was spending more and more time in bed, and due to our poor diet she had little chance to recover her strength. We were amazed one day when she told us that Fuji had started to bring her tit-bits of fish and other delicacies, that we had not seen for a long time. One day when he arrived with one of these offerings she thanked him and said he was very kind. She said she nearly fell out of bed when he looked coy and said "You my sweetheart, bye-bye my wife". We all enjoyed a laugh over this!

When Joyce and I were working in the kitchen and Fuji seemed to be in a reasonably good mood, we made subtle investigations as to the reasons for his attention to Maisie.

'You good man, you give our sick friend food.' This rather took him by surprise but he soon recovered.

'This man' - he always referred to us as men - 'plenty have got.'

Later we asked Maisie what she had that moved old Fuji to such admiration.

'Oh,' she said, 'I had that old trade box that I keep under the bed out one day and was sorting some of the things. Fuji admired my suede shoes, and the box!' Maisie had come over from the hospital in Kavieng after we had moved to Vunapope and was allowed to bring many of her possessions with her.

'I suppose he thinks I am not long for this world and he will inherit all my wealth!' It was a change to have a good laugh about Fuji and find he had some human traits after all.

Before the Club library had been locked away I had read what, under these circumstances, was a particularly interesting book by Philip Gibbs. It was a story about prisoners during the last war and the description of confinement in a German prisoner of war camp. The story bore little resemblance to life as we were experiencing it in Japan, though the behaviour and general outlook of the prisoners seemed rather like our own. The book was called *Wire Fever*.

Mr Gibbs described his characters, during their first six months of captivity, as taking a keen interest in sport and dashing wildly about the enclosure as though in haste to catch a train. This period most of us thought really did not apply to us, likewise the second one. That period, he said, was not so strenuous. "Violent friendships and equally violent foes were formed, many letters written and new uniforms ordered. Servants were hit for minor offences"! We found this account rather hard to believe, but of course it was written a long time ago and Germany in those days was considered to be a civilised country. However, the part about letters was intriguing since we were not allowed to write home, apart from that one letter from Vunapope, and we had never received any mail from home, either. We found this rather cruel, but put it down to a veiled form of torture - the price the Japs wanted us to pay.

We had no trouble identifying with the next two periods. The third: "It was almost impossible to express an opinion without causing an argument and one's mind ceased to function". The fourth: "Characters are put to the test, some go under and some just manage to keep their heads above water, while others rise to quite noble heights". My opinion of this last statement was that we had not gone under, were just an ordinary bunch, and just managing to keep our heads above water.

Spring, this year in 1944, brought us more than a relief from the bitter cold, Komatz and Basher disappeared from the scene and not even Fuji knew the reason for their departure. A month later we heard that Komatz had died and Basher went back into the Army. Our relief was two-fold. Our new guard arrived and we couldn't believe our good fortune. He was an elderly man, short and fat and more than a little senile in a happy avuncular way. We never bothered with his name we just called him Poppa San. Poppa liked to sing, so we would sing with him and teach him our songs. He had a little knowledge of the English language and disclosed the information that he was once a traffic policeman. He used to demonstrate by the hour how he'd *stopped* and *goed* the traffic. What we never found out was why he used these English words, but he seemed to be as happy with us as we were with him.

The guards were never with us for long and there seemed to be no pattern to their term of duty. These days we were on our best behaviour. We had no wish to lose this guard, yet we knew Fuji would do all in his power to get rid of him because he wasn't *bubbly* enough.

For the first time in seven months we were allowed downstairs to walk about inside the sea wall. One day when the weather was warm enough Joyce, Lik, Whytie and I let ourselves down over the wall and swam once again in the dirty waters of Tokyo Bay.

Army and Navy officials again visited the Club and inspected the rooms below and they took considerable interest in the now slimy swimming pool. Fuji was making himself appear important by giving us orders as he prepared a meal for them. Although we had seen him put on lunch for *big men* before, today he excelled himself. Fish appeared cooked in batter, with individual dishes of finely shredded vegetables quickly cooked in oil, accompanied by bowls of pink and yellow coloured rice. All this made our mouths water and perhaps we had been mistaken in thinking he was boasting when he said he had been a ship's chef.

As well as this hot food Fuji again produced the great Japanese delicacy *Sashimi*. I had recently read of Europeans acquiring a taste for this fish dish, which stated: "You could be in the heart of London and a longing for *Sashimi* might come over you and you would yearn to be back in the Land of the Rising Sun". It seemed to me that if the desire for this delicacy became so great, and as it seemed quite simple to prepare, why would you not prepare it for yourself in London?

When the feasting was over this day we did manage to scrounge a few left-overs. No *Sashimi* though, which of course started everyone exchanging recipes and conjuring up what we would do when we got our hands on wonderful, real food again. On these occasions it was particularly difficult to erase thoughts of mouth-watering dishes from our minds so we would write recipes down for

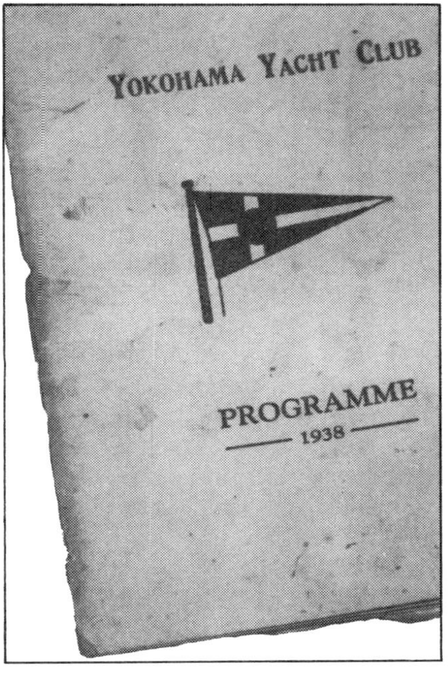

one another. Often they would be given as gifts for birthdays; among my treasured possessions is a gift of recipes from Joyce written in one of the Club's 1938 Yachting Programme booklets, issued to Club members yet somehow finding its way amidst this band of non-members.

War news, what little we could find, was encouraging with the Allies pushing up through Italy and the Americans very active in the Pacific. Although this was probably a played down version of the situation it was enough for us to make all-out efforts to see the papers.

Combined with the now warmer weather and all events, small and large, the future was beginning to look a little brighter.

Activity on the part of the Army and Navy officials turned us into detectives in the hope of obtaining some war news. Since the coming of spring the ice had melted on the grounds below and the fisherman gradually came back to the sea wall to cast their lines. We had not had an any real war news for some time and we kept a close eye on the fishermen - their bait was wrapped in newspaper! Many of these people, we had learned from Kimura, were shift workers from hotels and clubs and it wasn't unusual for them to have the *Nippon Times* (formerly the *Japan Times*). We didn't spurn the Japanese language newspapers either as they featured useful maps on the progress of the war. When the fishermen went off at intervals and left their lines we surreptitiously exchanged our old envelope-making newspapers for theirs.

Now that the ban on *sampooing* (walking) outside had been lifted, we began to fish also. We fished for seaweed with sticks and bits of wire and this was an activity of ours that had the approval of the Japs. The Japanese eat seaweed regularly with their rice and, although we never acquired the taste for it, we would eat it of necessity for its food value. When we became better acquainted with the fishermen we sometimes asked for the newspapers, which were mostly handed over quite readily.

In July 1944 we had been in Michael's *paradise* for two years. The *Chiefo* from the Foreign Office arrived on my birthday when the girls were giving me a party and told Kay we were to move today. Without any further information he withdrew in the direction of the kitchen.

This announcement of a move, although rumoured for some time, came as a real bomb-shell and there was the usual wild speculation though without the hope of our last move. There was definitely no interest in White Cross ships. We had long ago decided that the Japs regarded us as prisoners of war *not to be exchanged*. In relation to our group from Namanula I thought this decision would have had something to do with the fact that we were nurses in the employ of the Australian Government, and in the case of the missionary girls it is well documented that the Japs were indifferent to their Christian cause.

The birthday party broke up immediately and there was a scramble under tatami as bags and boxes were hauled forth, and in the case of Mrs Jones and Maisie a tin cabin trunk each. We were all ready, sitting around among our worldly goods - mostly rubbish - when two more men arrived from the Foreign Office. Immediately the *Chiefo* appeared from the kitchen with Fuji following on his heels, no doubt to act as interpreter if the *Chiefo* got bogged down.

'There is no reason at all why this man should not be able to get on with the "do good works and obey" routine speech,' Kay said. 'He has repeated it often enough.'

After about five minutes when nothing out of the usual had been said, one of the aides broke in.

'Remove your hats when the Chief is speaking.' The few of us who possessed headgear obeyed.

'No water at the *atarashii* (the new place),' was the next announcement. 'But,' he paused, 'plenty big gardens and food.'

We brightened considerably at this statement, yet it was difficult to equate 'plenty big gardens' with 'no water'. We made allowances for the Japs' muddled expressions and hoped for the best.

Half way through every year, since the Japanese had invaded New Guinea and changed our lives so dramatically, we had been uprooted for better or for worse. In 1942 the sea voyage ended in Japan. July 1943 found us packing in anticipation of boarding an exchange ship lying in the harbour at Yokohama, but we ended up at the headquarters of a police station in the city - a poor substitute and a bitter disappointment. Now it was the beginning of July 1944 and it was with very mixed feelings that we left the *boato* Club and set out for the country.

There was no expectation in our hearts just a 'get on with it' feeling; patience and tolerance were high on the list of things we had learnt in this imperfect environment. Though this move, at first, did not appear very promising and though the hardships were many, it was solely due to being in the country that we managed to survive and avoid outright starvation in the long year to come.

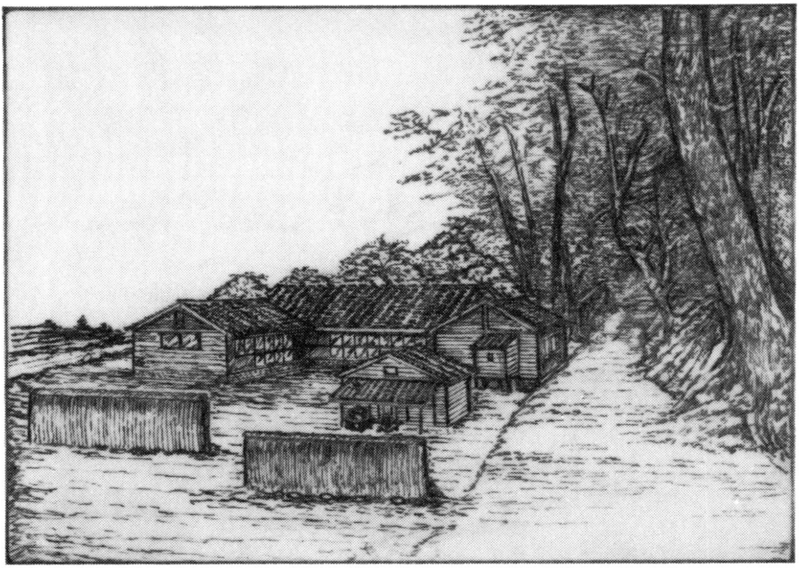

Our camp at Totsuka

8

TOTSUKA

Once again we boarded the *Black Maria*. The route today was westward through that part of Yokohama we'd travelled last year when taken on our sojourn at the police station. There was a dramatic change in the surroundings since then. Pavements had been dug up and planted with vegetable gardens, and motor traffic was practically non-existent. The city in general looked desolate, but when we reached the provincial area the striking difference promised hope.

Large clumps of pale bamboo stood peacefully among the endless changing pattern of remarkably small, cultivated fields. Tall pines overlooked tiny, thatched roof cottages indicating innumerable small holdings, and dotted here and there among them were peasant farmers in coolie hats. In the paddy fields country folk with bent backs diligently tended their precious crops of rice.

Looming in the distance along the road, we noticed a line of isolated barrack-like buildings. Was this to be our destination? We could see no sign of life as we drew nearer and felt something more than relief when *Maria* turned away.

Etched sharply against the summer sky the majestic sight of Fujiyama came clearly into view away to the south-west. It was inspiring to behold and we could see for ourselves that the Japanese had not exaggerated when they spoke with such reverence about their sacred mountain. The perfect cone of this extinct volcano rose gracefully from the lowlands, imperial and alone.

Just as our anticipation was soaring our transport halted in a decidedly neglected looking area. We tumbled out near a large building that was obviously a school. Nearby the squalid cottages and scrubby plants surrounding them made our previous euphoria vanish and we were quickly brought back to reality. Our driver and Junsa disappeared and were probably taking refreshments in one of the cottages while we were left to wonder if this would be our lodging. We waited around for nearly an hour in the hot sun and the schoolchildren stood and stared at us from under their straight black fringes. They gazed in fascination and scarcely moved; if they had ever seen European women before, I am certain our gaunt looking group would have borne them no resemblance. The Junsa finally emerged and waved his hands in the direction of this derelict area.

'This is the village of Totsuka. Follow me.'

With belongings in hand, we proceeded in single file up the hill. We followed the Junsa through tall trees where the path was winding and shady; for such an over populated country I was surprised to see large groves of trees about. On coming to a clearing a long low, wooden building with windows all around came into view. The rooms on the outside opened onto a corridor encompassing a courtyard, around which the structure stood in three individual sections. It was essentially Japanese architecture and was to be our new home.

'A nice summer residence,' Whytie said, 'and we won't be here next winter!' Whytie's subtle optimism had the immediate effect of a tonic.

Investigation of the building brought to light some aspects that were not altogether unexpected; after all, no water meant no sewerage. The lavatories at the end of the building were slits in the floor, under which were large concrete containers. We had experience with these 'vessels for personal use' at the Prefecture, so they came as no real surprise. We found no source of water at all inside the building, but outside, quite some distance away, stood a hand driven pump for drawing water, and standing near it was a very large wooden vat.

Situated a short distance from the back of the lavatories was a small wood and paper cottage. This dwelling, the residents and the 'lavatories' were to become our focus of interest during our confinement here. Incredibly these entities were to give us an insight into the life of the people of this rural area, the like of which, citizens of the Western world could never know.

By the end of the first day at Totsuka we had cleaned and scrubbed our quarters and discovered that the windows had easily removable frames. This was quite a good idea as, when removed, they allowed in an abundance of fresh air, although the air at Totsuka did not have the bracing fragrance of freshness. Another, not so pleasant, discovery was the presence of sputum mugs. These hospital mugs for spitting into are specially designed with lids for the control of germs. There were many of them lying around the grounds and under loose floor boards of the raised building.

'This must have been a Tuberculosis Hospital!' exclaimed Mary. This dreaded disease was one of the major causes of death in Japan.

During the afternoon a small battered vehicle arrived. We had given up thoughts of seeing our *tatami* again and this was a pleasant surprise, but not so the sight of that old devil Fuji climbing up the hill. Our one hope on being sent to the country was that we would be rid of him.

'Me watchman. All man go, me go.' His cunning greeting, displaying his broken discoloured teeth, left us exasperated, not to mention his persistent reference to us in the masculine gender.

'I just knew we'd never be rid of him, he'll be with us right to the end,' Joyce said disappointedly. Her prediction proved to be almost true.

As far as the nineteen of us were concerned we had a lot more individual privacy at Totsuka. Of the five separate rooms allotted, groups of four occupied the larger ones and Joyce, Lik and I shared a smaller room. The Junsa and Fuji had rooms off the kitchen at the other end of the building and the greatest advantage for us was that they were out of sight and hearing. Though we were entrapped here, Totsuka aroused a new awareness of hope. Hope clung as steadfastly as barnacles to a ship, and though it oft-times tapered, it would never leave us.

During the next few days we turned our thoughts to gardening. We placed into the soil the half-grown tomato plants we had brought with us from the Club, as well as our savoured pumpkin seeds, beans and sweet potatoes, known as *sashi* to the Japanese. However, we knew almost for certain that it was too late in the year for most of these vegetables to grow successfully. July was the middle of summer in the northern hemisphere and plants should be maturing now in readiness for harvesting before autumn.

To add to our tribulation coal for the fire and wood, which had to be chopped, was dumped in the village. It was one of our tasks to carry this from the main road up the hill to our lodging. Water had to be carried from the pump for use in the kitchen, and for washing; and up to one hundred buckets a day were necessary. They were not actually buckets in the true sense but wooden pails and quite heavy to carry before they were filled. In our present weak condition all this was tiresome work and there were always two or three girls just too sick to do anything now; Cal was so weak she was almost bedridden. Capping our woes orders came from headquarters that we were to dig trenches. This sign that invasion was anticipated was our one consolation.

The trench digging was to begin every morning at five o'clock until it was finished. Tools were produced and those fit enough got on with the digging. We had to be hauled out as we dug deeper we didn't have the strength to climb out and when the trenches reached about four feet deep we were simply too weak to lift another spadeful. Every day during the digging we asked Fuji for more rice with our breakfast, which was always at 7 o'clock.

'All right plenty inside,' he would say after he'd tipped an extra gallon of water into the already weak concoction. This gave us an extra drink but did nothing to appease the pangs of hunger we felt most of the time. Diarrhoea was constantly our worst complaint, interspersed with what we thought were recurrent bouts of malaria. We were so weak we could only stagger about and, with sunken eyes and general debilitation, we felt we had aged many years. I wondered what the toll on our health might be when we eventually depart this wretched situation and regain our former selves.

Obasan, which means honourable old woman, is the title bestowed on Japanese women from early middle age. Such was the title by which the small spry, bow-legged woman, who lived in the one roomed cottage right next to our *benjoes*, was known. She was in her early forties and her hair was piled on top of her head in the traditional Japanese style. Her bright darting eyes missed nothing and she carried herself with a dignity of manner so noticeably lacking in the other peasant women of this area, which set her quite apart. Her sense of repose inspired a quiet confidence in us and in time she became the central figure against whom we battled with what was left of our wits in our bid for survival. More importantly for our morale, she unwittingly became a great source of entertainment in our dismal lives.

Just after our arrival we were disturbed to see the body of a baby in the Obasan's house, a baby who had died quite sometime before. We were never able to find out whether or not it was related to the Obasan; in these early days we treated this woman like all other Japanese - with caution - and didn't ask unnecessary questions. For days the body was kept in her house and a Shinto or perhaps Buddhist priest - again we did not ask questions - bowed and prayed over the dead child. This man was swathed in yards of saffron coloured gauze and the rites he performed were interrupted by frequent cups of tea with the Obasan. The drinking of tea seemed normally to be conducted with a certain revered formality and on this occasion much more so. Other than the Obasan there appeared to be a scarcity of people attending the ceremony. On certain days young boys, chanting, carried a shrine around the house and one or two people dropped in from time to time. We were not able to find out if the ritual we had seen was usual prior to burial, but we assumed so.[1]

Very soon we did find out that there was a cemetery through the fence surrounding our quarters. After the baby had been buried for a few days and when there were no 'visitors' with us, two of the girls ventured through the fence one evening. In this burial place they found, on the fresh grave of the baby, a tin of milk. Nearby there were other flat mounds with food and cakes on them. This was a windfall. The powdered milk was a bit mouldy but the rest of the find, though a little dry and hard, was a real treat. In our depressed state of body and mind no one questioned the unearthly business of looting the graves of the dead for sustenance.[2]

The children of the village started coming around to stare at the big white women going about their chores, carting coal, pumping water and labouring in the garden. We must have been a rare subject for discussion among the village people whose only knowledge of Europeans could not be reconciled with this group before them, working, as they themselves had done for centuries past in their own struggle for survival.

We found ourselves living the humble life of the country peasant here in Totsuka, although these lowly born peasants had access to more food and were free to roam wherever they wished. We were now desperately hungry. The Japs had harvested their potato crop and the children carried potatoes around in their hands and nibbled this most prized vegetable as our children would sweets. Occasionally they threw pieces to the starving dogs which were always lingering about.

Being in captivity has placed great value on simple things once taken for granted when we were green-horns; the humble potato so readily available in Australia and New Britain now held a whole new dimension with us. Much has been reverberated about the plight of our ancestors in relation to their transportation across the seas in captive state; and, which should not be forgotten, the predicament of the Irish orphans. Now we knew from our own experience what the adversity of the great hunger of the 1840's, the Potato Famine, really meant to the Irish. In the difficult days ahead the production of the potato or its acquisition was our all-consuming passion.

The Obasan adopted the habit of popping in and out of our building at odd hours, especially when she knew the Junsa or Fuji would not be around. She knew no English, but our knowledge of Japanese which we trifled with in New Guinea had improved daily since coming to Japan. No one except Kimura and Fuji could understand us when we first came to Yokohama.

It was soon revealed to us that Fuji had lost no time in telling the Obasan of our cache of cigarettes, prudently saved from the Red Cross parcels at Christmas. The Obasan had never been seen without a cigarette hanging from her mouth! We had come to know that she craved tobacco as an addict craves drugs and tobacco of any kind was in very short supply. By this time we had also come to know, that it was an offence for the Japanese to trade in food with the 'prisoners', so caution and diplomacy would need to be exercised on both sides. In this quandary, we wisely left it for the Obasan to make the first move, which was not long in coming.

The room shared by the three of us was nearest to the house of the Obasan and one night she made an appearance through the lavatory door. Without making a sound she slid open our door and dropped a bundle on my futon. It was full of knitting and sewing materials.

'The village people' gestured the Obasan, 'had takusan (a great quantity) of this stuff.'

In return for knitting and sewing they would give us *takusan* of potatoes. The Obasan was something of an actress and we had little difficulty in understanding her meaning. For her role as intermediary we rewarded her with some precious cigarettes.

Every one was delighted with the scheme and immediately became active. The gifted knitters, Whytie, Joyce, Kay, Greenie and Chris set to work and formed the Dai Nippon Expert Knitters Ltd. The limited, they said, was added to indicate that there was a limit to what could be done with such a mess of tangled wool on improvised knitting needles of bamboo. It had to be washed, sorted, cut and twined together again before anything could be made with it.

The knitting venture went well, the village people were pleased with the patterns and quality of the products, and we received a good supply of potatoes. Our hunger pains waned and sleep was easier. Then one day we were struck a severe blow when the villagers asked for their wool back, which meant that no more potatoes would be forthcoming. This turn of events upset the knitters as they really thought their customers were content. Surprisingly, one day at the pump the villagers threw pebbles at them!

A few weeks later on a very cold morning the cause of the problem was revealed. The culprit appeared wearing a *kimono* over which she also wore a very smart jersey, and the girls immediately recognised their work. The Obasan always collected and delivered the finished garments! Later when the local people found out about her duplicity they arrived with potatoes and vegetables for us.

It was somewhere around this time that Dan came into our lives. He was the *benjo* or lavatory man and we naturally began to refer to him as Dan, the *benjo* man. We thought of him as the male counterpart of the Obasan since he was almost a match for her when it came down to the business of barter.

Dan always arrived in the morning, jogging between the shafts of his square wooden cart, his open coolie coat flying. He wore blue trousers which fitted like tights and came half way down his bare legs. Sometimes he wore a fur cap covering his ears and looked so comical that he could have been dressed in disguise for a character part in a Japanese folk play. To proceed about his business Dan backed his cart up to the concrete containers under our lavatories, removed a small door to gain access and, by means of a long handled scoop, filled his wooden tubs. In the rural area the sides of the roads were lined with containers into which Dan and his colleagues emptied their tubs. The stench was terrible!

The operation on our *benjoes* took place almost on the doorstep of the Obasan's living room and it was soon apparent to the interested observers that Dan was on very friendly terms with her. He always took a break from his work when she was 'at home'. He would skip the few steps across to her house and bow before stepping onto the matted floor; having no shoes to remove he carefully cleaned the soles of his feet on the straw mat outside. We never ceased to be amazed at the paradoxical make-up of the Japanese especially when it came to every day hygiene. Dan never washed his hands before his morning tea sessions with the Obasan!

The plants in our garden were showing no signs of progress, which was not really surprising as there had been little rain and we were forbidden to use water on them. As "the world's best gardeners" the Japs knew how to get around this problem. I had never heard of compost neither had I heard, nor had any of us, of fertilising as practised by the Japanese. While we were labouring in our garden one day the Obasan approached to cast a professional eye over our efforts.

'Dame, dame!' she exclaimed disapprovingly. Her message was clear, we must use the Japanese method of gardening - apply *benjo*! After the initial shock registered we realised that the vegetables we had eaten since coming to this *paradise* had been nurtured in this manner. As the days crept by our vegetable garden persisted on being uncooperative. Should we *benjo* or perish with hunger?

There were among us, the "I wouldn't ever do that" anti-fertiliser group, impervious to reason. It did not take long, however, for hunger to win out and our slogan arose: No *benjoing*, no crops. A new problem faced us regarding Dan. We would be encroaching on his territory, this enterprise after all was his livelihood. Like so many converts the die-hards became over eager and in order not to encounter Dan they got up at first light to use the scoop before he arrived. This tool on closer inspection was found to have holes in it causing it to leak badly and, worst of all, the handle would not stay attached.

The project proved to have more pitfalls than the scoop! This fertilising venture caused pests to multiply a thousandfold. Slugs and snails started eating the plants almost as soon as they began to show signs of growth. The enthusiasts suggested that we set up a roster to keep an all-night vigil on anything that flew, crawled or wriggled. The old-timers, Lik, Joyce and I, thought this was taking things to the extreme and, fortunately, our suggestion to carry on as usual was agreed upon.

When eventually reaped our small crop was commented on scornfully by the Japs, nevertheless, it supplemented our deals with the Obasan and did give us a feeling of well-being, how ever slight. This addition to our diet lessened the diarrhoea though it was not enough to improve our muscle weakness. Our distended stomachs and lumpy tissue of the hips and thighs stayed with us.

There was one day when I was elated to find pigweed growing among the grass. This used to grow well in the outback of Queensland and I was amazed to see it in this cold climate. Cut up and added to the tasteless rice mixture it made a pleasant change. The main disappointment was that although we searched for more we could not find enough of it to be beneficial. Its sacred healing properties as claimed by the ancient Greeks may have given strength to Cal who was very sick now.

There were so many smells around Totsuka and we had no way of getting out of their range. They followed us inside when we closed the sliding doors, seeped through cracks and penetrated the useless masks of rag we wore over our noses.

When we first arrived we thought all odours were the aftermath of Dan's daily business activities. However, after further forays into the burial grounds we formed a different opinion. On investigation of a newly filled grave we found that the body, which was not contained in a coffin, had the barest minimum of soil covering it. Since this was insufficient it was no wonder the stench was overpowering. We did not know the reason for burying a corpse in this way. The cemetery was out of bounds to us and we had no wish to arouse ill feeling with an inquiry, but we assumed the graveyard had been in operation for generations past and perhaps an acute shortage of plots caused the graves to be used more than once. After the findings of the tombs, as we called them, we had to admit that it was unfair to blame Dan for every stink that assailed us.

In pre-war days globe-trotters to Japan brought back stories about the cultural diversities of the Japanese, particularly of their spiritual leanings towards the after-life and their bathing habits.

"The Japanese are devoted to cleanliness". This virtue, proverbially next to Godliness, was the unanimous opinion of those mostly casual observers, a judgement made on seeing the many communal bath-houses throughout Tokyo. Bath-house buildings were easily distinguishable by their tall towers penetrating the skyline. Fuji had told us in Yokohama that centuries back too many fires were caused with accidents to wood-fuelled water-heaters in the fragile Japanese houses and, in order to prevent them, it became law that no commoner's house could have a private bathroom, henceforth the public bath-house came into being. Whole families attended the bath-house to cleanse and refresh their bodies and as time went by this gathering of the people, relaxing in the steaming hot water, became a pleasurable social habit which continues today.

Here in Totsuka in early autumn the Obasan took control as organiser of the bath to rid the locals of accumulated dirt and livestock after the hot summer, the livestock being fleas and lice. She hustled us off to her house one afternoon, when Joyce and I, Whytie and Kay were pottering about forlornly in our garden plots. The vat-like wooden tub, which was apparently the only one of its kind in the village, had been placed outside the Obasan's house and was to be used as the communal bath. A metal pipe was fixed at the bottom and came up inside at one end, a partition divided this pipe from the bather. Several empty buckets were standing near and the Obasan directed us to fill the tub with water.

The Obasan bustled off to gather anything combustible she could find to add to the wood already stacked. She deposited the fuel next to the bath and judging by the pile she managed to build, while we pumped water, it was going to be a long session. People from the village drifted in with bundles of food, which they left on the

Obasan's *tatami*. They whispered, and watched in awe this singular event of foreign women preparing the bath for their provincial kin.

The sun was setting and there was every indication that it would be a warm autumn evening. When the tub was nearly full the Obasan waved us away to our quarters and got on with her fire lighting. We, undaunted, lost no time in taking up a secret vantage point to view proceedings.

The scene was about to move into the second stage with the Obasan mistress of ceremonies. To coax the flames, she puffed and blew vigorously through a short bamboo tube; fathered by green bamboo twigs and bits of bark, swirling smoke soon clouded the scene. Squatting on her haunches in the hazy evening light the Obasan conjured up a vision of a medieval sorcerous concocting a deadly potion.

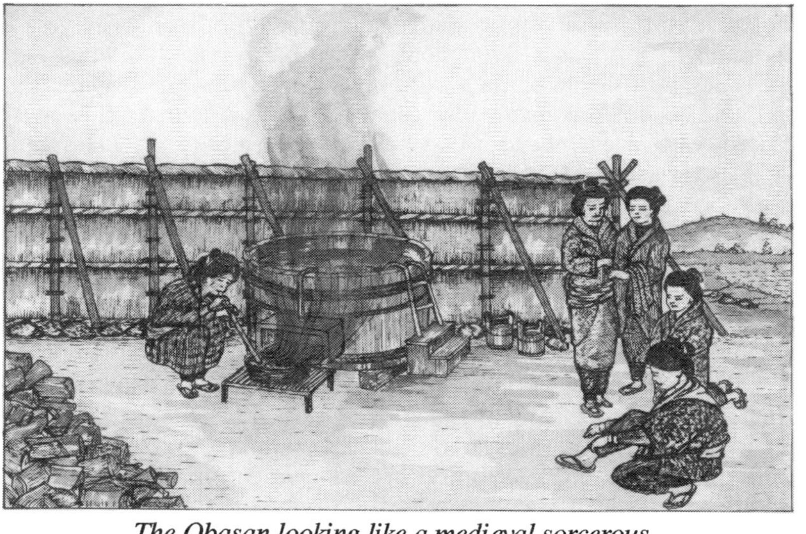

The Obasan looking like a medieval sorcerous

A fine fire soon blazed and all was set for full steam ahead. As small groups began to arrive there could be no doubt about the evening being a social event - we were surprised at the large gathering. A few of the women busied themselves cooking over the *hibachi* in the Obasan's lean-to. The Obasan was more fortunate than her neighbours in having a lean-to outside her cottage for cooking purposes.

As the steam began to rise from the water our Junsa stepped

forward. Being the most important person present it was his privilege to be first to take the bath. Stripping off his clothes he helped himself to a pail of hot water and soap. He scrubbed vigorously and helped himself to more water to rinse away the soap and dirt. Our guard had completely lost his identity as he mounted the small stool and stepped cautiously into what appeared to be almost boiling water. We were pleased to note that the body must be thoroughly soaped, washed and rinsed before entering the bath.

Mothers and aunts started delousing the children while awaiting their turn. This chore was simple in the case of the boys. Their heads were closely shaven with just a tuft of black hair left standing upright above the forehead. The style made them look very comical but was, undoubtedly, a sensible arrangement under the circumstances.

When the Junsa finally emerged from the hot water he was as pink as a cooked lobster. In a very relaxed way he seated himself cross-legged, completely nude, on the Obasan's matted floor and was offered a plate of steaming sweet potatoes and a cup of *sake* from Tomari, the Obasan's daughter.

Half way through the proceedings Dan arrived. Apparently anticipating a cool evening he had added a short coat of some recently skinned animal to his apparel. When Dan's turn to take the bath came round his image, resembling something between his usual character from folk theatre and tonight an Eskimo trapper, vanished as well when he shed fur coat and cap.

What struck the interested, though now rather disappointed observers, was the solemnity of the occasion. The bathing habits of the Japanese, as described by visitors to these shores, sounded like a jolly frolic, something like a dinner dance in the nude! Whytie, who had been observing the scene from a crack in our lavatory wall, said they looked as though they were attending a wake.

'Back home in Hay we had more fun than this on a Sunday School picnic, followed by a dip in the Murrumbidgee.'

'You mean you went swimming in the nude?'

'Well, not quite, on a Sunday School picnic,' she said on reflection 'but we did have some fun!'

As the night air grew cooler some of the not so hardy bathers ran up and down in an effort to keep warm before joining the increasing circle on the *tatami*. No towels were produced though a few of the women draped colourful pseudo scarves around their necks and shoulders.

At intervals throughout the long evening someone would visit the observation post and report on the progress of events. Close to midnight the final observer declared that the entertainment was nearing an end.

There was now a complete circle of men, women and children on the matted floor of the Obasan's house; the surplus had overflowed to the ground below. It was a very sombre gathering, with some squatting, and others sitting cross-legged, all with skin the colour of blushed peaches after immersion in the very hot bath. The only activity was among the workers, the women who had yet to take the plunge and were busy supplying steaming sweet potatoes and small cakes to the bathers. All were served green tea in small bowls with the exception of the honoured guest who was still receiving his tot of *sake*. The entire event appeared to be steeped in reverence and unity. We wondered if it might have been the abstention from alcohol which accounted for the absence of frivolity among the bathers.

The Obasan had stoked energetically all evening and was sweating and weary. It was now time for her to take a well deserved turn in the bath. After half an hour had lapsed we began to wonder if she had fallen asleep, but at last the tough old girl emerged. There had been no one stoking for her and the water must have been cold. Briskly brushing off surplus water, she approached our room near the entrance. She had come with an invitation for *Minna* to take the bath. We declined with thanks!

'Ah So!' She hissed and gave us one of her sly sideways looks. 'The Goshus are not clean people like the Japanese?'

We tried not to laugh before she padded off to join her guests. She would no doubt have a well earned glass of *sake*; no tea for her on this occasion.

After a short time of living in this rural area several myths about the servility of Japanese women, their abiding patience and gentleness, became revealed as not altogether what the symbolism suggests. I thought this had particular reference to the older women who could, and often did, retaliate when sufficiently provoked or considered they were. On reflection, our first example of this was that matriarch at the Bund Hotel, Mrs Saito, who unequivocally controlled her household, and there was the woman guard, Moricame, who asserted authority over Fuji for the short time she was on guard at the Yacht Club.

It is true that Japanese women did prostrate themselves and bow deeply when greeting their lords and masters; their position is one of natural inferiority. They worked side by side with the men in the fields yet when the demand arose men would prepare and cook the food. Here in the country women worked hard, carting and chopping wood, carrying water and doing all the jobs necessary in a rural community. So too, did pioneering women in other countries and from our view of it, Japan could not be classed as belonging to the enlightened twentieth century as we know it.

The status of women was not a myth in Japan, but a tradition. Ethics and proper behaviour for women are laid out in a Japanese manual, Onna Daigaku. Women are at the bottom of the social hierarchy and are taught that their lot in life is obedience; obedience to the father in childhood; obedience to the husband in womanhood and obedience to the eldest son in old age. Having learnt this from Poppa San we understood more about the time at the Bund when we were made the equal of Japanese men by officials from the Foreign Office. This concession bestowed on us must have been almost a courtesy with curious respect to our position as Australian women, prisoners in Japan and devoid of family!

When the Obasan was out of cigarettes she smoked a small pipe with a lid covering the bowl; it looked like 'silver'. We had no idea if she filled the pipe with anything other than tobacco but we did have some doubts on the days when she was particularly *genki* (happy).

A brawl was not an uncommon occurrence in the Obasan's house and, always in control, it was she who sent hunks of wood flying from her fireplace while the men sat silently waiting for the storm to pass. At times the Obasan's brawls with Dan were particularly lively.

It was our belief that Dan was aspiring to be on intimate terms with the Obasan, however, judging by the off-hand way she usually greeted him we came to the conclusion that she thought him her social inferior. After I learnt that Dan kept chickens as well as running his *benjo* business he surely must have *takusan* of money and, consequently, would make her a good husband. My suggestion outraged her. She spat on the ground to show what she thought of the idea. She had an *ichiban man* (meaning a very good husband) in Tokyo, she said. This was the first we had heard of this paragon; we never saw him and she never mentioned him again.

Joyce and I and the Obasan were in the kitchen one day when Dan arrived looking very chirpy. He greeted us and walked over to the Obasan who was smoking her pipe. She was obviously out of cigarettes and not in the best of spirits. She sprang out of the chair and pulled off his cap. He spat on her hair and grinned at us, demonstrating his authority. The Obasan pounded him with her fists and he lost his jovial air and delivered a *karate* blow that laid her on the floor. A big jar of salt fell on top of her. At this stage Joyce and I left the scene, however, we did return later to gather up some of the salt, a commodity in short supply.

A few days after this incident Dan was sitting with the Obasan chatting happily, sipping green tea and eating cake; the scene portrayed a very convincing peace offering. Following the event of the 'bath' the Obasan had told us that the Japanese hold spiritual faith in the ritual of tea drinking, or *O-cha* to name it in Japanese politeness. We thought that this ritual was really no different from our own meaning of having tea with friends, but with not quite the conscious formality. The tea ceremony in Japan symbolises a manifestation of harmony, reverence, purity and tranquilly.

Since our internment we had come across articles in the newspapers about the Japanese devout love of children, which was fundamentally true. It is just as true for all people of all nations to have the same natural love, yet children might sometimes be neglected through ignorance and poverty. Many children in Japan wear a charm against accident and an identification disc, should they become lost, a mixture of superstition and practicality which seems to be part of the Japanese disposition. In Totsuka the poor hygiene and general physical situation could be attributed to what we would consider slum conditions. Children had lice in their hair and clothing, their diet consisted chiefly of rice and potatoes and at no time did we see them drink milk or eat eggs. They sometimes had fish with their rice, but rarely green vegetables few of which were available in Totsuka. The outlook was not promising but the children always seemed happy.

From our reckoning it appeared that the Obasan had her fair share of children and grandchildren and, without doubt, she loved her three year old grandson, Noburo, dearly. He was a happy, normal child who thrived on his diet of rice and potatoes and toddled around nibbling the sweet *sashi* in his stubby little hand. His eyes seemed always half closed and his nose constantly running.

One morning when we were standing outside in the feeble late autumn sun Noburo came toddling up to his Grandmother's house; he was just tall enough to haul himself onto the matted floor. He removed his *geta* as usual, and when he couldn't find anything to wipe his feet on he picked up one and then the other and licked his soles as a kitten does its paws.

We thought this ridiculously funny and when we told the Obasan about the theatrics she looked at us with feigned indifference.

'Of course.' she said. 'Noburo is a clean Japanese child.'

She made it apparent to us that this was not an unusual performance by Noburo.

One day the Obasan went off on what we referred to as her 'business trips' and left her 'silver' pipe on the low table near the sliding doors. Noburo was asleep nearby and on waking he rubbed his eyes and slowly moved towards the table. He looked amusing since the Obasan had cropped his hair closely and left the tuft, unclipped, sticking up on top of his head as was done to most of the little boys. Noburo picked up the pipe, opened the lid and, after taking a long draw, made the motions of blowing smoke through his nose just as his Grandmother does. When he saw we were watching he carefully shut the lid on the pipe and laid it back on the table. He sat on the mat, put the soles of his feet together and clasped his hands over his fat tummy. Noburo gave us an impish grin and in this pose he looked the image of a carved miniature Buddha.

These small diversions in our boring lives helped us forget our plight and made us feel normal. They filled the ever present emptiness and eased that "when will all this end" tension in our minds.

In the autumn of 1944 we were undergoing a particularly bad time and relied a great deal on trading with the Obasan. Our rations consisted of only tiny bowls of rice and carrot tops; the ever recurring scourge of diarrhoea was at its worst. This was the period when the summer crop of potatoes was finished and the *sashi*, the lovely sweet potato, was just beginning to appear, but not in our garden.

I was still in possession of my nursing shoes, the compulsory low heeled lace-ups. They did not interest the Obasan personally nor any of the other villagers apparently, until the cold weather set in, which it did very early this year. Snow fell early as well and proclaimed a foreboding testimony to the commencement of winter.

We were restless as the evenings grew colder and wondered how we would be able to sleep with ever increasing, gnawing pains in our stomachs. One night there was a gentle tap on the window. We jumped up to find the Obasan motioning us to come with her. In her lean-to we were confronted by a few village people and a man whom the Obasan introduced as her brother. Many times she had hinted that she had a brother who was a 'wealthy farmer' and had *takusan* of *sashies* and other delicacies. He wanted to see my shoes and I lost no time in producing them. The Obasan beckoned us closer to the fire while her brother thoroughly examined the shoes. With much hissing and haa-ing he inspected the soles and seams minutely. He all but turned them inside out and without trying them on to see if they fitted declared his verdict. 'Yoroshi,' he said, which, we all knew, meant in English that he was well pleased with them.

'Well done Hall Shoes!' I said to myself. 'Wear your crown with propriety!'

Sighs of relief came from our group, though one thought did reluctantly cross my mind: What a sight I would look arriving home with a distended stomach, lumps and bumps on my thighs, minus a few teeth and to cap it off, bare feet! Of course nothing really mattered at this time but the result of the bargaining.

The Obasan, her brother and all the other guests joined in the talks that went on and on. The Obasan gave us a small *sashi* each as we waited hopefully for a decision. Finally she announced that over a period of one month we would be given seventy pounds of *sashi*, bean curd, peanuts and soya sauce. For her brother and of course herself, as well as my shoes, they were to receive *takusan* of cigarettes, soap and boot polish. The two latter items were much sought after and the Obasan would have no trouble trading for more cigarettes with the soldiers at the barracks, not far away, in exchange for the soap and shoe polish she had artfully acquired.

The final details of what was considered a good deal by us came to an end with much bowing on both sides. My shoes were no doubt the first pair of real shoes the Obasan's brother had owned; he proudly tied them around his neck with the laces, shuffled into his *geta* outside the Obasan's house and departed.

Joyce, Lik and I were feeling quite excited and reported to the others on what we felt was a favourable business agreement. A few of the more nervous girls brought up the subject of Sunlight and Nugget. These two products, received in our Red Cross parcel, had undeniably undergone some changes in quality and quantity since leaving Australia. As the need for bartering became apparent we had employed our wits. Sunlight was boiled down and some chalky shampoo powder added, which we bought with the paltry *sen* given in payment for knitting the little bags at the Club. This project resulted in six cakes of soap from one. A similar thing was done with Nugget. When one tin was mixed with Japanese face cream and various dyes it ultimately filled a much larger tin.

Later when we were all in our own rooms the Obasan made one of her silent sideways entrances. She had come to tell us that her brother would deliver the *goods* every night and she would cook them in her *hibachi*. This arrangement seemed to suit everyone and was a pleasant change from the endless conflict of opinion we had come to expect now over almost everything, how ever trivial. As a group of prisoners we were small in number to be confined for so long together and being in such close quarters gave vent to constant paltry disagreement. We were from three classified organisations of our profession and tended to remain within our own secure circle; probably this alone was the greatest cause of dissent. However, we were always staunch and unified in real crisis.

Snow continued to fall and we dreaded the months ahead. We made many tracks in the snow every night when a representative from each room visited the Obasan's lean-to, to collect the unwashed, unpeeled, saltless *sashies*, and no gourmet meal ever tasted as delicious or could have been more appreciated. The peasants of Japan could not sustain life without the sweet potato, it was symbolic of the quest for survival. It represented to them life itself and now played that role in our own struggle. Joyce, Lik and I often called up visions of the *kaukau* growing wild in the tropics and we couldn't help wondering how many of our counterparts all over the world might be paying homage to this humble vegetable as we were.

Over the period of the deal there were many disappointments for us. Startling sirens would cause the damping down of the fire in the cookhouse; sometimes the Obasan would have unexpected visitors or perhaps she had a sufficient quantity of cigarettes on the particular

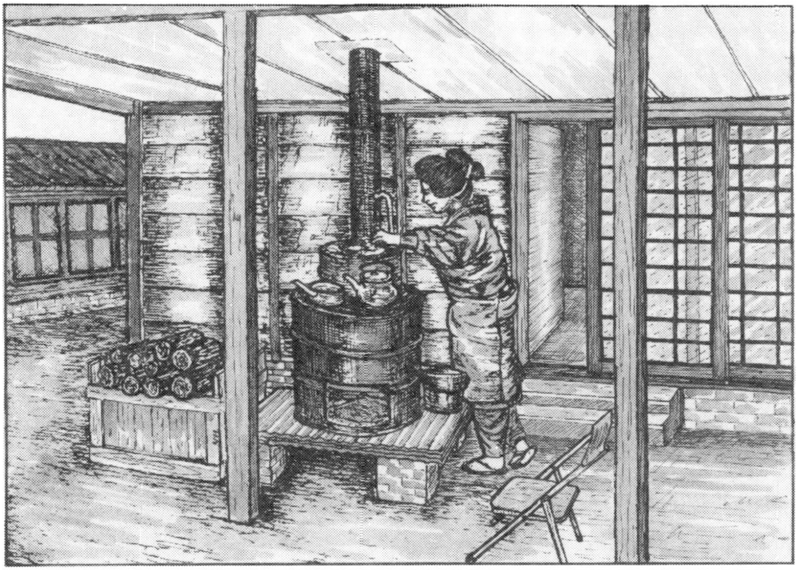

The Obasan cooking sashies

evenings we were destined to go without. On these nights we would be dismissed with her favourite utterance.

'Ima nai, ashita.' Not now, tomorrow.

These curt words dashed our hopes and reduced us to supperless, sleepless nights while we waited for *Ashita*. The Obasan, however, usually kept her word and would arrive next morning with our cooked sweet potatoes often covered in ice! *Ashita* always came and though it was an unknown quantity we placed blind faith in it, faith in the words, *ima nai ashita*.

The fact was often discussed that the Obasan never bothered to conceal her bartered cigarettes from the ever present Mori, who had come to Totsuka after us. We came to the conclusion that she not only had the police under her thumb but Mori as well - we could not be sure about Fuji, but we were certain that she supplied those she wished to influence with foodstuffs and *sake*. Whatever bribes she used it was obvious the Obasan had things all her own way and for this we were thankful. We often had a quiet giggle when musing the venerable lady's Shinto heaven paved with *hakos* (boxes) of cigarettes and lined with bottles of *sake*!

Several days after the shoe deal had taken place the Obasan became jittery and paid us a visit to find out where we stored our goods - as though we had much choice! She was worried that *big men* might visit Totsuka and search our quarters and if they found any *sashies* she would lose her head. She omitted to say what was likely to happen to us!

Our supplies of anything valuable or illegal were hidden in the ceiling where a loose board was easily removed. For some reason the Obasan did not approve and advised us to put them under the *tatami*. Later, to reassure the old girl, we put an empty box under the bed and told her *shimpai ga nai* (not to worry). We found it rather amusing to think that the *big men* would be too dignified to stoop down and peer under a bed like alarmed spinsters.

Another worry reared its ugly head, the ever increasing invasion of rats coming in from the fields. Rats the size of small cats wakened us in the night; we fought them off as they ran over our beds and chewed at our hair. We were really alarmed when we heard the loathsome creatures scurrying in the ceiling and from then on we kept sticks as bludgeoning weapons beside our beds. We knew that they, too, must have been truly starving when they nibbled our manufactured soap. Joyce, like us all, was afraid of the rats, but she was beyond doubt more afraid of snakes. Lik and I, with some trepidation, assured Joyce that these rats were big enough and savage enough to cope with any snake.

The snakes lived under the floor and came up through a hole; a hole that could not be covered successfully and so worried Joyce. We reminded her that it was her Irish ancestors who had persecuted snakes and quite probably that was why she had such a fear of them. Kay actually killed a snake one day and was angrily castigated by the Japs. They relied on the wretched snakes to control the rats! Following this incident Joyce no longer had any faith in our assurance.

Just as the Obasan had done with the village people's knitting, the cunning old girl did with the goods her brother brought, as part of the trade for my shoes. She watered down the soya sauce and deducted *sashies* for her own use. We decided the best solution would be to waylay her brother when he came around again and request that delivery be made direct to one of us. To this he readily agreed with many smiles and bows. The Obasan undoubtedly had a guilty conscience and attempted to make amends by saying that the Japanese were *doroba nai* (not thieves). To restore our previous harmonious relations with her we said that the thought of the Japanese being dishonest never entered our heads. We knew we were back on our former footing when she cordially replied *Yoroshi*. It was unusual for a Japanese to be as forthright as the Obasan was with us; but then she was different in many ways which we rather enjoyed.

We ate a good many of the sweet potatoes raw and the general opinion was that they tasted like apples. Some days old Fuji would sleep in the afternoon and we seized these opportunities to go to the kitchen and cook a few *spuds* to supplement the ones from the Obasan. The possibility that she might not comply with her part of the bargain, for whatever reason, always threatened, and we strived to prepare ourselves for any potential setback which could deny us our food.

We scrounged for food wherever we could and on one of the days when Whytie was rummaging through the rubbish heap next to our building she unearthed a picture of the Emperor! Fearing we would be blamed for this desecration of the Son of Heaven she wiped the surface clean and stood the picture against the wall. Later of course it was found by the Junsa who, after much bowing and saluting His Imperial Highness, went off to see the Obasan who would be asked to explain. We were unable to find out how the picture came to suffer this indignity and in the meantime we were concerned for the Obasan. We ought not to have worried on her behalf, she came out smiling from her interrogation, though not so her daughter Tomari who was crying. We heard nothing about the incident and were not questioned over it, and we knew it would have to remain unsolved. We doubted if even that renowned sleuth Sherlock Holmes could have solved this insult to the God Emperor Hirohito.

A few days after this episode the Obasan came running up the hill from the direction of the village.

'Minna, hayaku!' she screamed while grabbing a bucket and pumping furiously. She ordered us to bring more buckets and do likewise. Following the Obasan we staggered down the hill trying not to spill the precious water and when she stopped abruptly we nearly fell over her. Instead of a raging fire we found a heavily laden cart, and between the shafts lying on the ground was an old ox. The poor animal looked as though he would never rise again but, after giving him a good drink and splashing him with the remainder of the water, we eventually coaxed him to his feet. With a resigned look he went wearily on his way up the hill; an animal's life in Japan is not a happy one.

Ill-treatment of animals passed unnoticed or was taken as nothing unusual, and to knowingly allow animals to starve did not seem to disturb the conscience of the Japs. In spite of our own experience we could not understand this insensitive attitude. Kimura, the Club steward, would have seen his dog starve to death, but we decided it should be put out of its misery. From what we had seen so far adults did not interfere when children displayed heartless traits. Kenjita, the Obasan's teenage son, thrashed his dog brutally one day for walking on his garden and his mother and other Japs thought nothing of it. They did not rebuke him when he caught birds and tied their legs to a long string, letting them go several times, all the while pulling the poor birds back to the ground until they were finally exhausted. This sadistic behaviour bothered us very much, but we were helpless to do anything about it. Little wonder that these people gained an infamous reputation for acts of barbarism during this war.

At Totsuka it continued to be our job when on kitchen chores to take the Junsa's food to his room. Breakfast was always rice topped with pickles and this, accompanied by green tea, would be his sole daily meal if vegetables or bean curd were not available. Children from an early age are accustomed to such food, so it did not come as a surprise to us that the Japanese took powders for stomach disorders and suffered from indigestion and intestinal complaints in later life. It could be said quite truthfully that the Japanese are a dyspeptic as well as a myopic race.

Pickles in Australia that our mothers made bore no resemblance to the Japanese variety. In Japan vegetables are shredded, chopped or sliced and placed in wooden vats with layers of salt, and left to ferment. Stone fruit is usually left whole and treated in a similar manner. The result is a hard, heavily salted pickle ruinous to the digestion. Soya beans are placed in vats with wheat and salt and the resultant bean curd, *mezo*, is nutritious, and to the hungry not so bad, and definitely not as hard on the digestive system as some of the other Japanese concoctions. Salted plums, pickled cucumbers and grated dried fish are greatly relished by the Japanese. Soup made from bean curd and served with leeks is another delicacy and quite palatable, though we were never offered this beneficial dish.

Over the fence, near the pump, a few pumpkins were growing wild and as we hadn't spread our seeds there we found this amazing. When we went out for our water supply for the night we would take an extra bucket and eventually a few small pumpkins found their way into the ceiling above our rooms. When we ran out of food and the weather was very cold, as a last resort, we would eat raw pumpkin. After a while it made us very nauseated and we tried to 'keep off' this diet until an opportunity arose to do some cooking, but this was a sad mistake. A few freezing nights later when we needed our pumpkins most we discovered a black watery mess. Sometime after this we acquired some two-feet long *daikons* which again went into the ceiling, but this time we kept a cautious eye on the weather. The *daikon* is a white vegetable of the radish family and grows to an unusually long length. It is very popular with the Japanese, but it tasted revolting to us so we made an effort to pickle it.

Joyce seized a tinful of wet bran mixture from Fuji's pickling cask; we split the *daikons* lengthwise, as we had seen done, brought out the wooden pail and a pickling process was put into action - or so we thought. We had forgotten the essential ingredient, much additional salt, of which we had none. Days later we awoke to a new odour, sour, fermenting *daikon*. After facing the problem of getting rid of it we closed down the pickling factory as a bungled effort.

On the first day of November we were astonished, and filled with joy, to hear air raid sirens wail; although there was no raid in the vicinity it was a sure sign that our Allies were active. It lifted our spirits and, quite understandably, seriously upset the Japs. The Junsa and the Obasan were very quiet and made no comment, but in the kitchen old Fuji was full of fight and fury and chased Joyce with a knife. Joyce said she had never moved so fast in all her life. From now on when sirens started up we thought it wise to keep well away from the Japs. Air raid precautions were acted upon and Dan emerged as a warden sporting a warden's pixie cap. As the war seemed to be almost upon us, excitement mounted, and we were very anxious to know the course it was taking.

The Japs were glued to their newspapers, which were well illustrated with extensive maps of the Pacific area. From these *Courier Mails* we decided that the Americans were conducting offensives in the Pacific from Guam, in the Mariana Islands, and must be in control of the Philippine Sea. This meant that Guam had been taken back from the Japs and possibly other island strongholds in the Marianas group. With this Allied victory it should only be a matter of time before retaking the Philippines where the papers were showing obvious activity. And then it would be Japan![3] Needless to say our expectation of the end in sight heightened.

Meanwhile, the population in Totsuka had been piling on clothing for well over a month now and continued as the weather got colder. They were completely enveloped in clothes, and weighed down with so many layers which probably did not do very much to keep them warm. From our observations of the community it seemed that they seldom changed these layers during winter and we wondered if the lice and flea population might not be hibernating in them.[4]

One night the Obasan came in to discuss a potential deal with us and immediately began hopping about scratching herself. She put her foot on my futon, rolled up her trousers and proceeded to pluck at the seams. I wondered how many were getting away into my bed and Joyce said I looked horrified. The Obasan gave me one of her sideways looks and said these were *Goshu nomies* - Australian fleas. They were not Japanese fleas, they were too *okii* (big); she thought this a great joke. Strangely we did not have lice in Japan, but there were times in the summer when we got little sleep with the outbreak of fleas. The fleas caused such irritation that we looked as though we had measles and to compensate we cut our hair as short as possible.

At the beginning of 1943 the Japs had made a *presento* of sufficient material to enable us to make a pair of slacks each. This mixture of wool and some other fibre was reasonably warm and proved hard wearing, but now, serving its third winter and being our only garment, it was threadbare. On our diet of watered down rice mixed with a sort of sticky flour, and no heating of any kind a serious look at the months ahead promised gloom. With some ingenuity we found a way to line our clothing with pockets of newspaper, used as insulation in an attempt to keep us warm.

The weather was very cold and most days and nights we sat

around too weak to bother with anything. We had very little to say, each dwelling on her own personal thoughts in the solitude of despair. Over the years our families and our lives had been discussed so many times that we knew each other intimately. I could picture Joyce's sisters as if they were my own; she, unlike Lik and I, had no brothers and we willingly shared ours with her. Liklik came from eastern Queensland - not as far into the Never Never as I, but a thriving sheep farming area.

The three of us had a lot in common, it was as if we might have grown up together. We had no way of knowing if our brothers were fighting in New Guinea, but we felt pretty certain they would be. Joyce's Bill had been posted to the Middle East quite early in the war and of course she had received no news of him since our capture and did not know how the destiny of war had placed him. In my mind thoughts presented the image of a jig-saw puzzle which had been tackled over and over again but gave no satisfactory result. There were many gaps where pieces were missing and I so looked forward to the day when each piece would fill its special place.

On one of these melancholy evenings, after our potato deal had come to an end, Joyce, Lik and I were sitting around as usual when there was a tap on the window. Much to our astonishment one of the girls from the village was outside holding a bag dripping with blood.

After some negotiating and no questions asked as to the origin of the *presento* she settled for three packets of cigarettes. The Obasan, she said, knew nothing about this deal and as direct bargaining with the village people was unusual we thought it necessary to be discreet. The mess confronting us looked to be the intestines of some small animal and cooking it was going to pose a problem. Hungry as we were we could not eat it raw!

This would not be the first time we had devised methods of illicit cooking. At the Yacht Club in Yokohama we had used the electric plate salvaged by Kay during our raid on the boat-house. At Totsuka our method was more primitive. We used tins of various sizes which were fuelled by pieces of anything we could find; cooking in this way took several days. The main problem faced with this offering was to prevent the savoury aroma, that was now so rare as to be unmistakable, from being identified by the Japs. Somehow all ended well and when one of the girls produced a small pumpkin the stew was transformed into a gourmet dish. Even without salt it was given the stamp of approval. We were truly aware that we had come a long way since that first night in captivity when a real gourmet meal, made by the nuns at Vunapope, was our evening fair. How much further could we go and when was it all going to end, I wondered.

Snow covered the ground and wind rattled the building. When the wind blew from the north it piled up under the roof above our frail ceiling. A hole in the roof was a constant source of worry allowing snow to build up above us and we were anxious to be rid of it before it melted. Poor Lik, she did come in for some dirty jobs since she was the smallest, therefore, the only one able to squeeze through the narrow opening in the boards. The accumulated dirt must have been a foot deep up there and when she came down she looked like a chimney sweep.

The winter of 1944 was our third winter in Japan and decidedly colder than we had experienced so far. Here in the country it did bring out a picture postcard beauty of this land of contrasts. Towering Fujiyama, in a mantle of snow, formed a magnificent background to the countryside. The chestnut trees, pine and cedar, their branches covered in snow, stood as guardians of the pure white ground. Winter snow hid the squalor and smothered the odours, and thatched roof cottages added to the illusion that we could have been looking upon the scene of an English countryside.

This perception of beauty around us could not fortify us from the reality of the bone-chilling temperature. The dreaded season had really taken hold and we had to pool our scant resources, and our wits, to find solutions to hunger and cold. To the problem of cold there was no solution; we would just have to endure as best we could. To the problem of hunger we sought one solution for the time being and our target was Dan.

Tentative suggestions had been made by Dan in the past about some children's clothing which, strangely, was included in our Red Cross parcels. When it came to trading Dan had always been wary of poaching on the Obasan's territory and nothing had come of attempts to secure deals with him. There was a difference now, we were desperate.

Our opportunity presented itself when the Obasan went off early one morning on another of her business excursions. Keeping watch, we waylaid Dan as he came in with his cart and buckets. After some small talk he began to discuss his three young sons and we, very timely, brought out the children's clothes. Khaki shorts and shirts had no bartering value in the past and we thought this was because they were the stamp of Western society and therefore an unacceptable substitute for the ubiquitous pyjama-like tops and pants of the Japanese youngsters. We couldn't understand why such a rural character as Dan would suddenly want them for his boys, but put it down to the capricious behaviour of the Japanese.

As well as the clothes Dan asked for a packet of tobacco. We asked for forty eggs, and without a change of expression Dan yelled, 'Baka!' He finally agreed on nineteen eggs, one for each of us, and cakes twice a week for a month.

Dan came knocking at our windows when all was quiet at the Obasan's residence and it was no problem to jump from under futons to take delivery of sticky cakes wrapped in newspaper. They gave us acute indigestion but what they lacked in nutrition they made up in bulk. One thing which pleased us greatly was his nocturnal delivery, it meant that Dan did not arrive with these goods tucked away among his fertiliser buckets!

Cal had been really ill for sometime and was now bedridden; it was doubtful if she could survive the cold winter. One day a Japanese doctor came to see her but, of course, he had nothing to tell us that we did not know already. He offered nothing either, in the way of food or medicine and he might as well have stayed away. We knew she had Tuberculosis and all we could do was make her comfortable and give her as much nourishment as possible which, under the circumstances, was hopeless. Since coming to Japan, in our scavenge for sustenance, we had always eaten scraps left over by the Japs, our need left us no option. Tuberculosis germs were everywhere and in our debilitated state the risk of catching this highly contagious disease was considerable.

The peasants at Totsuka were cut down to meagre rations of rice and fish. An article in the *Nippon Times* stated: "Everything must go to the Army; Japanese people must make sacrifices".

'Makes it sound as though these poor wretches lived the life of Riley at the best of times,' Goss said sourly.

On a particularly dismal morning Lik, Joyce, Whytie and I were trying to concentrate on a card game when Kay put her head in the window.

'The Junsa says we are to come at once there is a man from the Foreign Office here.'

Throwing aside the enveloping futons we rose with a speed seldom in use these days and followed Kay down the passage. This man was a stranger to us and we lined up and bowed without being told to do so. After the routine introductory, "You must be grateful and do good works", he proceeded to hand out a few small parcels.

As we unwrapped the parcels there was stunned silence when silk socks, cotton briefs and short sleeved shirts and handkerchiefs were revealed. The items were all men's wear and our hearts descended to our *geta* at the sight before us; they were probably destined for a camp in Singapore or elsewhere in the tropics. We bowed and thanked the "kind gentlemen" as they departed, giving us no indication that they were surprised at the contents. Later, when our disappointment eased a little, we found it quite amusing and wondered how men in camps in a sweltering climate would react on receiving a parcel of women's woollen underwear.

At last! At long last, the real thing was here! Sirens screeched a violent warning to the Japs on the 24th November, but were to our ears the crescendo of an orchestral composition one could never tire of listening to over and over. Bombs dropped in the vicinity of Tokyo and Yokohama and the evidence was irrefutable; war had come to Japan. We heard nothing about the results of this attack, but our excitement was extraordinary and all we could think of was tomorrow. Optimism gushed from us as we sensed the war was going our way and with newfound enthusiasm we celebrated a late Melbourne Cup, cheering confidently that next year our bets would be placed on real horses.

However, all this excitement provided little warmth from the cold. Mori told Kay that we were to be issued with futons, but these never arrived, which surprised no one. The people at the Foreign Office had a habit of promises that were never fulfilled, yet the Junsa was seen nestled cosily under a new padded quilt one morning when one of the girls took in his breakfast!

Mrs Jones was able to supply blankets for the sick girls, Cal and Maisie, and life would have been virtually impossible for them without the extra warmth. Maisie was very weak most of the time, and Cal's strength of spirit in her crisis truly amazed us. There seemed no doubt that both her lungs were infected and how she managed to survive the severe cold we did not know. Being hungry and cold is difficult to bear, but to be hungry, cold and as sick as Cal presented a tragically different story.

On some nights when walking the passage to stimulate heat, Joyce Lik and I glimpsed with envy how effectively the Obasan went about keeping warm. There seemed to be little privacy in the Obasan's house. Large sliding doors were always open and gave no domestic seclusion and the comings and goings of visitors, of which there appeared an endless stream, were a source of fascination to us.

In her one roomed house there was a large cavity in the centre of the floor which remained covered over during the summer months and at the beginning of winter a *kotatsu* was placed in it. This heating apparatus comprised a wooden box with a burner, sand was put in the base of the box and fuelled with anything combustible, but mainly coal. An iron frame can be placed over the top of the *kotatsu* for the suspension of a kettle and cooking pots, for the dual purpose of cooking, but the Obasan used her *kotatsu* solely for heating. Her cooking was done on the *hibachi* in the lean-to.

On the nights the Obasan's guests stayed over futons were taken from cupboards lining the walls and spread on the floor. Everyone with the exception of the Obasan lay on the padded quilts with feet as close as possible to the heat so that the bodies formed a fan around the *kotatsu*. Finally, the Obasan would close the sliding paper and wood doors and presumably complete the circle on the floor.

The Obasan's younger children got up early on freezing winter mornings. Still dressed in the clothes in which they'd slept, they washed their hands under the pump - when it wasn't frozen - grabbed a handful of rice from the *hibachi* and trudged off through the snow to school. The children fended for themselves in winter as they did in summer and they must have been driven to despair at times by hunger and cold.

One day the Obasan's children were digging in the snow around the trees and, after collecting a few pieces of twigs and rubbish, they lit a fire on the higher ground by scraping it clear of snow. Other children joined them around the feeble flickering flames and one small child was crying miserably. The scene reminded us of Dickens' England, which was never so much under discussion as at this time.

'It only needs a girl with her feet in the snow selling matches,' I said to Dorothy Beale who was also watching.

'Or singing carols under windows and waiting for a penny to drop from above,' said this leader of the missionary nurses.

During December people began trickling out of the city, particularly at week-ends, bringing possessions to store in the country. These were not impoverished people but more affluent citizens of Tokyo and Yokohama, many were Foreign Office staff and important Government officials. As this building was one of the largest in the community many of their boxes and crates were being stored in rooms and courtyards at the rear. With all this activity we could only assume that the Allies had begun their offensive on Japan and that the November raids had caused this alarming impact.

As Christmas approached and deals had come to an end our food supplies were extremely low. While in Yokohama we had read a book by a Frenchman who stated "A meal should be light and contain nothing to paralyse thought". None of us agreed with this statement these days, our diet was light yet our thoughts were paralysed; anchored on food, awake or asleep, the getting of it and the eating of it. Among the nineteen of us we had only a few cigarettes left and nothing else with which to bargain should an opportunity present itself.

There was little Christmas cheer in our camp; the days were bitterly cold and the wind rose and whipped the top of the snow. There was nothing to do; cold and hungry, we huddled together in our rooms in silence. Our room was at the end of the building and one morning Joyce, Lik and I heard talking further up the passage. We stirred restlessly and shortly afterwards Kay appeared.

'The Junsa wants about six of us to go down to the road and pick up some boxes. More stuff from the Foreign Office I suppose, they certainly are making a store house of this place.'

Heads down against the wind we followed the guard and when we were almost at the roadside he held up his hand.

'Matte (wait),' he said. A few minutes later a lorry pulled up and started off-loading strong cardboard boxes. We all came alive at the same time.

'They've got Red Crosses on them!'

No one waited for an order now, as with renewed strength we surged forward and loaded ourselves up like coolies going to market. It was the 21st December, so near to Christmas and we were overjoyed.

From near starvation to what seemed like mountains of food in just a few hours was mind-boggling. Everyone was talking at once and the din almost reached hysteria level as we opened the boxes containing tins of jam, milk, coffee, sugar, raisins, prunes, chocolates, butter and meat. And last but not least for the trading potential they offered, cigarettes and soap. When the excitement died down a little each room group decided, more or less according to willpower, to spread this bonanza over as long a period as possible. The non-perishable goods said the more strong minded should be kept. With a good cigarette supply we might be able to get *sashies* and so struggle through the winter without too much privation. We had not yet had a taste of real war on Japanese soil and could not be expected to know the overwhelming effects of refugees on the poverty stricken rural community!

As Christmas day drew near it was certain to be another White one, for which there was little enthusiasm. Next year it would be sun, sea and sanity and on this subject we were in complete agreement. Privately we all knew, that which ever way the war went, under another winter of these extreme conditions we would find it impossible to survive.

On 24th December 1944, Christmas Eve, the sun shone brightly. The snow covered peaks of Mount Fuji glistened in the distance, inspiring hope and banishing unpleasant thoughts of gloom. Everywhere could be heard happy forecasts of how we will celebrate this time next year - not of *now* but *tomorrow*. Without a doubt the present euphoria was related to the state of our stomachs.

'An appropriate background for Christmas carols,' Chris said as she hung the now rather tatty decorations of other years.

On Christmas day we wrapped small parcels of sugar, raisins, chocolates and tea in the only paper available, toilet paper; the fact that we were each giving and receiving almost the same gift made no difference to the pleasure involved. The only one singled out for anything special was Cal. We all gave to her what we knew she would be capable of using and eating. A much appreciated gift of sweet potatoes from the Obasan added to our tinned Bully beef and made a real Christmas feast. From the kitchen came a gift of bread which had been off the menu for a long time. Later in the afternoon the Obasan lent us her kettle and we rounded off an almost happy day with bread and jam and real tea. This, after all, was a most promising Christmas.

The festivities were short lived however and we faced the realities of the cold winter anew; we had never experienced such low temperatures. Our rags and tatters, when put outside to dry, froze, almost as soon as they were hung on the line; they looked like the bizarre shapes of a string of scarecrows. Ragged as our clothes were they were never thrown away, and any material left over from patching them was used to repair the futons, which were not only falling to pieces, but had taken on that unhealthy damp mustiness when cloth is permeated with grime. By now though, we could almost ignore smells of any kind and except for the girls with malaria, we had a good idea too that we must be immune to most infections, which was one blessing.

The Japs said that this was the worst winter in twenty years and we did not argue with that. Snow lay feet deep on the ground and the pump, our only water supply, was almost forever frozen. These days we wore the same sets of clothes almost continually. The two old smelly futons issued to each of us in Yokohama provided very little warmth and in the evening we huddled together on our straw mats. At various intervals through the night we tramped up and down the passage in our quarters in an endeavour to keep our circulation going. Oh! How I longed for the hot, dry heat of the outback or the sweltering days of the tropics.

The local people seemed to have gone into hibernation and the Junsa spent a great deal of his time crouched over the *hibachi* keeping warm and playing *Go* with visitors who wandered in from the cold. Fewer visits by the village women were made to the pump - which was likely to be frozen anyway - and the Obasan was not entertaining as frequently as before. As the Obasan was our main source of interest we found ourselves missing her 'goings on'.

There was very little to stir the imagination these days, but when we saw the old water pump, looking like a Victorian figure in a broad hat and wide skirt, we thought this quaint improvisation warranted applause. These straw garments were devised to keep the water from freezing; rural farmers sometimes wore garments made of straw to protect them from the cold and rain. The idea of clothing the pump may or may not have been successful; on most days no water was forthcoming until the afternoon. In our building we tried storing water in wooden pails but they invariably leaked and became firmly attached to the floor, frozen, and when we picked one up one day the bottom was left behind. Joyce and I soon gave up morning ablutions altogether though Lik persevered for a while. When loud smashing and banging woke everyone up she was persuaded to give up too and go unwashed like the rest of us.

'The days are long enough without getting up at the crack of dawn.'

9

TOTSUKA - WAR

The New Year of 1945 brought an end to our third year of captivity. Quite out of the blue Mori informed us one day that we could expect to be bombed soon, people were already leaving Tokyo and Yokohama. We knew only sparsely populated cities in Australia in comparison with Tokyo's eight million population and Yokohama right next door with about half that number, and it made no sense that a few fleeing could make much difference. Where would they seek refuge anyway in these overcrowded islands of Japan? We were reminded of a similar dilemma the local inhabitants of Rabaul had and although on a much smaller scale we had our doubts about the safety of this strategy.

'Heavy fighting going on in the Philippines.' Mori seemed anxious to tell us as many snippets of news as possible. Perhaps he had chosen to get the war in the right perspective and unload his worries on to us, as safe outlets. We were certain the Japs had lost the fight and it would be just a matter of time now. We were just as certain the war in Europe would have ended months ago and found it hard to believe that it still dragged on; information which Mori reported with a hint of satisfaction.

I thought we had gained some insight into the contrary ways of these enigmatic people, but an eye-opener came our way when Mori handed Kay an order from the Foreign Office.

'Here you are girls,' she said, 'this is going to take you weeks to sort out.'

The gasps were audible as Kay read the incredible order. Mori shuffled, looked confused and padded silently away.

'"Write out all the gold and jewels in your possession and do not conceal anything or you will be punished".'

'Surely everyone at the Foreign Office can't be crazy!'

'Imagine wasting time on this sort of nonsense,' Joyce said.

'Perhaps it was meant for some of the more affluent internees if there are such people in this country.'

Only Mrs Jones had something of value, her wedding ring and wristwatch. After some consideration it was agreed that it would perhaps be too facetious, as much as we were tempted, to tell the truth and list: One pair of earrings for pierced ears, round brown buttons with pins, one necklace of 'silver' *sen* threaded on silk supplied by the kind Japanese and 'left over' from knitting those small bags for them and, on inspection, no gold found in teeth.

February brought increasing air raids and stricter Government control of food. *Sashies* were available now, but even the Obasan seemed to be observing the restrictions regarding dealing in foodstuffs; at least temporarily. She told us that there was plenty of food for soldiers, but little for civilians and to give food to us was *dame dame*, very bad, and that once more she would be in danger of losing her head! This was her favourite when she wanted our sympathy.

Of course, as usual it was not long before the Obasan forgot these dire warnings. These days she was reduced to smoking her long-stemmed silver pipe and, having been hooked on American tobacco since our arrival, she was undoubtedly finding the local stuff hard to take. We gave in to temptation when the Obasan approached us with a new proposition; the warmer weather was months away and our savoured Red Cross supply of food was shrinking. The Obasan would give us a moderate supply of *sashies* for an inflated amount of cigarettes, but she decided it would be too risky for her, this time, to cook the spuds. She definitely got by far the better deal, however, we consoled ourselves with the fact that we did have a good quantity of cigarettes available and that this would be our last winter here anyway. This optimistic outcry was usually voiced after an air raid.

The Junsa spent most of his time in his room studying the newspapers. Maps in the papers showed a great deal of American Naval activity all about the Philippines. Because of the intensity of the Junsa's interest it must mean the Americans and our Aussies were gaining ground, getting closer to us, closer to our freedom.[1]

Would *Ashita* soon be here? What a morale booster! How many prisoners were in Japan and did they have access to newspapers? Were other nurses captured and spending their time somewhere in Japan? The Japs must have taken many prisoners when the islands fell; where were they all? These questions we'd asked ourselves many times but would only know the answers with the coming of *Ashita*.

As the exodus from the cities increased so did Dan's status in the community. Daily he went about his business, plodding to and fro between the shafts of his cart, hauling baggage up from the roadside and transporting vegetables and wood, in general doing good works. There was still his *benjo* trade but in these busy times this trade seemed to be just a sideline wedged in between more prestigious duties.

One morning I was on kitchen chores when Dan appeared between jobs to take *O-cha* with Fuji, who was in a good mood and seemed to be basking in his friend's new status.

'He big man, take sick man in cart go doctor, go market, bring box, big man from Tokyo.' How he managed with just his cart I couldn't imagine.

'Bombs come put out light.' This last reference was to Dan's status as an air raid warden. There was no doubt that Dan the *benjo* man had become a prosperous and notable citizen.

Early this month Mori ordered us to clean out the trenches. These were the square holes we had dug soon after our arrival in Totsuka. These places for the purpose of refuge had become a dumping ground for all kinds of rubbish and were probably alive with vermin. We thought these holes were more likely to trap than shelter, as any close bombing would cause this building we lived in and the Obasan's house to collapse within minutes smothering the occupants of the hole. No one would be interested in our views so we kept them to ourselves and got on with the clearing. We had hardly any energy and certainly no enthusiasm for the job and it took us a long time. We knew there would be no *presento* in the way of extra food either.

Near the anniversary of the fall of Singapore the long-awaited, long-hoped for air raids began in earnest. Bombardments increased daily and changed our lives completely. Gone was boredom and despair and our squabbling attitude. Instead of *next year* revitalised spirits claimed *soon*, and our major objective was to stay alive, an especially difficult goal in the relentless cold of a winter that seemed to drag on and on. With the renewed bombing, hope was no longer elusive and our frailty strengthened miraculously.

One day an air raid ended in a fierce dog-fight overhead and several Japanese planes were brought down in flames. After this battle a formation of little planes with turned-up wings flew at great speed just over the tree tops and caused the windows to rattle; some of the girls said they saw stars on the wings. We were certain now these were fighters returning to their carrier. They were the fastest aircraft we had ever seen and we estimated that they must have been flying at a speed of at least four-hundred miles an hour. Witnessing the Allies at last, at such close quarters, was the most awe-inspiring and morale lifting milestone since our capture.[2]

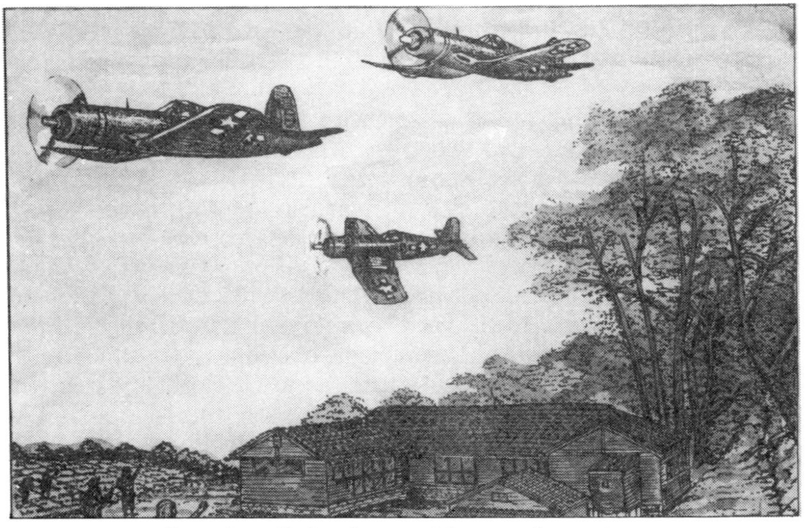

Corsairs - little planes with turned-up wings

At Totsuka there was a great deal more activity among the locals following these raids. Soldiers from the nearby barracks held manoeuvres in the pines and bamboo clumps, camouflaging themselves with branches. Schoolboys drilled with wooden guns and shrill commands rent the air as they lunged with their mock bayonets.

An anti-climax followed the uplifting effects of the February raids, when those little fighters with turned-up wings flew over our heads. A lull in the raids brought disappointment, but I suppose it was unrealistic to expect action to be around us all the time, just because we were close to Tokyo. We held fast to the belief that elsewhere in Japan assaults were being carried out by our boys.

Encouraging news came unexpectedly when Mori brought in the *Nippon Times* and showed us the bulletin that read "For the first time the enemy has soiled our sacred earth with his muddy boots". By reference to the maps we assumed that the tiny remote island of Iwo Jima, with its strategic airfield, was the sacred soil in question. We could get no detailed information but were thrilled to know battles were being fought and, we assumed, being won so close to us. We were filled with anticipation and it was impossible for us to disguise our joy, so we made no real attempt.

Food supplies in the village had reached an all time low with an influx of refugees; our food had reached an all time low as well. The optimists thought that the Americans must surely know that the country was on the verge of starvation and would sue for peace.

'The Yanks can't come before spring anyway unless they are equipped with skis.' When this opinion was expressed, by some of the more pessimistic, no one knew that at this very time the Allies were winning the war in Europe under similar conditions!

'Well, we might be out by the end of the year yet, if we last that long.'

'We will last that long!' The optimists never wavered.

We went about our chores shovelling snow and retrieving bits of bark and twigs we had hidden previously from old Fuji's prying eyes. We heated water in our empty meat tins until at last the snow began to melt.

With the melting of the snow in March the first signs of spring were upon us. Water trickled down the mounds where vegetables had battled for survival last summer. Heads of hardy wild flowers and the first green leaves of spring shimmered in unexpected sunlight. Mrs Jones had a brief moment of despondency when she told us of the beautiful flowers appearing in spring in Alaska. Most of us were amazed, our vision of Alaska pictured it forever covered in snow.

With the exception of Cal, we languished outside most mornings trying to make ourselves believe we could get some heat from the sun. It shone so brightly over this Land of the Rising Sun, presided over by the Sun Goddess, but no warmth came from it.

No matter how often we heard an air raid siren wail it never failed to start off that prickly sensation of skin and hair and rumbling in the stomach, especially when empty. Today was no exception and within minutes of the sirens sounding as we waited silently and expectantly two huge planes appeared. No more followed these giants as they headed in the direction of Tokyo leaving in their wake swirling white vapour feathers silhouetted against the blue above. There were no explosions and soon the all-clear sounded.

Excitement abounded and for once we were in agreement. It was a reconnaissance visit and pamphlets were released with peace proposals. We just had to wait. These days Mori could not keep information to himself for long; he seemed to impart bits of information just to make himself feel important. However, we were to be disappointed on this occasion, Mori remained in a room with the Junsa, and the Obasan kept out of our way also. As the afternoon wore on a few of the village people came at varying intervals to the Obasan's house.

Something big was going on. That was the verdict!

We kept out of sight on the other side of our quarters and prodded the heaps of rubbish under the melting snow but found nothing edible.

'There's been a terrible smell close-by since yesterday,' Whytie announced.

'What's new about smells?' we wanted to know, but Whytie wasn't to be put off and climbed over the fence while the rest of us kept guard. The last time she had visited the burial grounds there was no food offering for the spirits of the dead or for the stomachs of the living and again today she returned empty handed.

'It's only a dead rat.' Whytie announced so dejectedly that we were almost amused. As we wandered back to our building a cool breeze was stirring, thankfully banishing the bad smell.

'You know there's something strange about today,' said Oldroyd. 'The sun is shining and it looks and even feels like spring, but there is no life in the trees.' Oldroyd was a believer in omens.

'You'll be looking for elves and fairies next,' I said, but did not admit out loud to having a strange, sinking feeling myself. As evening approached the wind was curiously gathering strength, showing signs of an unsettling night, adding further despondency to the anti-climax of this morning's excitement.

'Perhaps we've been expecting something dramatic after those raids last month,' said Chris, who was never one to display a discouraging outlook. 'This morning's visit by the Americans might bring some action yet.' At all times throughout our internment we could rely on Chris and Whytie to be cheerful and optimistic.

That night, 9th March 1945, it was difficult to sleep with the fury of the wind howling around the building. It whipped through the ceiling and disturbed the snow which began to drip. There was much muttering about springtime in the country as we shifted our beds. The ongoing effort of removing the snow had proved trying for poor Lik and we had given up the undertaking long ago.

A penetrating siren woke the group of restless sleepers. No one knew what the exact time was when the alarm startled us, but our guess was close to midnight. Everything seemed to be happening at once and we rushed to the windows facing east to see Tokyo burning.

Sweeping flares penetrated the heavens and illuminated scores of low-flying planes dropping their cargo with obvious accuracy. Totsuka was about fifteen miles from Tokyo and we had a clear view of the action in the sky. Not one word was uttered, as almost in disbelief we were absorbed in concentration; it was as if we were viewing a dramatic scene captured on the screen of a Hollywood movie. Flames were caught in the swirling winds and danced upward, turning into fire balls feverishly feeding upon themselves. Explosions tortured the air and the shocking scene took on the spectacle of a volcano in violent eruption.

Scores and scores of, what were to us, magnificent American planes kept coming in waves. There were agonising gasps when a huge bomber plunged earthwards in a flaming spiral to disappear in the holocaust below. The radiance issuing from the fires, caused by this fierce bombing, so lit up the area that here in Totsuka we could read newsprint.

The dreadful phenomenon being enacted reached a peak when a lone bomber, like a terrorised spider, was exposed in the giant web of searchlights. Beams of light cris-crossed the heavens hunting their target as it flew with all its might seeking escape in the darkness. As the suspense went on, hour after hour, there was not a light or sound in the village or on the nearby highway. We quite openly breathed audible sighs of relief when our gallant Allies, on completion of the night's sortie, flew into oblivion like the closing scene of a real movie. But in Tokyo the drama on the ground remained. No longer gasps and squeals from us, we began to discuss what all this would mean and what would be the outcome.

During 1941 we had listened to radio reports of the devastating bombing of London and other major cities in Europe. How remote it had all seemed from that distance of thousands of miles away; even the shock attack on Pearl Harbor was hard to visualise. We held a vivid memory of the invasion of Rabaul, yet this disaster witnessed in Japan was frightening beyond imagination; the number of planes and amount of explosives they dropped was inconceivable.

We could see no sign of the Japs around. What their thoughts must have been as they watched their hallowed city showered with bombs from a mammoth enemy force was not something we wanted to think about too much.

The all-clear sounded just before dawn. Fires no longer exploded, and the sky turned from flaming crimson to impenetrable black. Shrouding the horizon to the east, blanketing the glow of dawn, were clouds of dense smoke carried by the wild wind that had helped whip the flames into last night's inferno. The acrid smell of smoke took over from yesterday's scent of spring and reminded me of the aftermath of a destructive Australian bushfire and it was not hard to visualise the anguish these people would be suffering.

This morning we all stayed willingly indoors. Sometime ago we had given up discussing what would be likely to happen to us following a circumstance such as this. The discussion always provoked futile argument and, on most occasions, our views were usually opposite to the reactions the Japanese portrayed. The devouring of food was driven from our minds this morning, only unanswerable questions occupied our thoughts. How would the Japs react to the assault on their capital? How had our men in the camps fared? Did the Yacht Club get hit? And worst of all, for the consequence it would have, was the Emperor's Palace bombed?

There was no sign of the Junsa, so Kay said she would find out what was going on.

'Good luck!' the rest of us said, without much conviction.

'We must just place our faith in God,' Chris said, and no one had anything further to add; not even Tootie (Daisy Keast) who in any past crisis always voiced the opinion that she expected to be shot!

It was a long time before Kay came back looking relatively calm.

'Mori's daughter has come from Tokyo, his house was destroyed but his family are safe,' she said, and went on to tell us that Fuji had left for Tokyo to find out about his family.

'Mori was very upset but otherwise appears quite composed and polite,' Kay continued. 'He said thousands of people are streaming out of Tokyo and a great many of them have nothing left except the clothes they are wearing.'

'And I'll tell you something else that Mori said which will lift the weight from your minds. The Imperial Palace *wasn't* bombed!'

During many previous discussions we had addressed the possibility of the death of the Son of Heaven, by the Allies, and unanimously agreed that this would definitely spell disaster for us. Their Emperor was a God to them and we knew, instinctively, his death would see the extermination of all prisoners held by the Japanese.

That afternoon Kay appeared with the *Nippon Times*.

'Mori gave us this copy, it's all about last night's raid.'[3]

"America and Australia are strong and powerful now" was the general theme in the newspaper. "We are very sorry for the destruction the Americans have done to our country, it is very cruel".

In the days following the burning of Tokyo there was no end to the stories of horror recounted in the *Nippon Times* and they were corroborated by those who had first hand experience of that night. Countless survivors, now homeless, were flooding into country areas and inadvertently adding to the burden of the already hungry, peasant population. There had been little instruction given to the people of the city about emergency evacuation.

The Sumida River was a magnet that drew thousands to its banks that night only to find that almost everything except the water blazed. Piers and warehouses were infernos through which the escapees had to find an opening to reach the lighters lining the river banks. Those who managed to push off in these small craft had no easy task as they paddled their way to the centre of the river; floating corpses with their clothing still steaming obstructed the passage. Closer to the banks frantic swimmers thrashed at anything moving in a desperate effort to save themselves. If these people believed in hell they surely must have thought that this was it. Eerily, the water reflected the flames on the blazing banks and the river flowed like a ribbon of blood.

The raid that night concentrated on industrial areas along and around Tokyo's Sumida River. The Japanese were introduced to intensive bombing early this year but were ill prepared for what happened on the 9th March. The American Super Fortresses carried incendiary bombs, which generated fires almost impossible to extinguish and the fickle wind that night was in collaboration with the Allies. On impact, the force of the wind caused the incendiaries to rage beyond expectation through the streets and channels of Tokyo, like tornadoes devouring everything on their crusade of extermination. Thousands of factory workers lived close by in their fragile wood and paper homes; nothing and no one in the path of destruction was spared. The people had been ordered to build holes under their houses as a place of shelter during a raid; no large public air raid shelters were constructed.

Reports in the paper told how people suffocated and burned to death in these inadequate shelters. Most of those who escaped into the streets were already severely burned when they ran towards the river and many did not reach their destination. They wore heavily padded capes with hoods which were designed to protect them from bombing and subsequent fires. With these incendiaries the capes smouldered slowly and the wearers were not aware of being alight until burns were actually felt on the skin after the incendiary fires had eaten through the thick fabric. There were babies who suffocated on their fleeing mothers' backs before it was known such a shocking thing could happen to the infant snuggled within.

Seeking safety from this hell on earth and the intense heat that was generated, the people fled to the parks and gardens lining the river bank. As the masses swelled, panic arose and those nearest the banks were forced into the river. Thousands of bodies were reported later to have been fished from the Sumida estuary.

The many canals in the area were crossed by small bridges which collapsed under the weight of those seeking refuge on them. Most of the escapees drowned clinging to one another in the narrow waterways.

When the river widened into Tokyo Bay salvation was at hand for the survivors of this holocaust and, although ships and wharves were alight, there was space to breathe in the fresh air from the sea.

Almost every Japanese that we'd been in contact with from the city had lost his home and among them was old Fuji.

Kimura, the former club steward from Yokohama was also among those homeless. When he arrived in Totsuka one day he told us that he had lost his wife and children in the Tokyo raids. Japanese have a strange habit of giving a false laugh when relating tragedy. Kimura acted this way when talking to us, but when he walked away he was crying.

I thought it a strange twist of fate that a little over three years ago those of us from Vunapope had witnessed the blitz on Rabaul from almost the same distance as Totsuka is from Tokyo. That saga marked the beginning of Japan's proposed conquest of Australia and the Pacific; this blitz on Japanese soil marked the end of that outrageously ambitious plan for a *New Order in the East*.

A few days later an astonishing assumption was revealed in the *Nippon Times*. "Although the Allies now have superior strength they lacked the uplifting and purifying Japanese spirit of *Bushido*. Due to this spirit and the country's preparation to fight a twenty-year war, the Japanese will emerge victorious".

Japan was so desperately short of food now. It was amazing that politicians in a devastated country could still attempt to delude the people with such idealistic outpourings. How could *Bushido*, the spirit of the warrior, save them now. It was impossible not to feel sympathy for the millions of simple people who had been plunged into a war, causing them to suffer so much and probably be the chief losers.

The six-hour long battle of 9th March ushered in a new era as far as we were concerned. We had made the wrong conclusion yet again. The increased activity on the part of the Americans, surprisingly, brought us a great deal more freedom as we were not the focus of attention any more. As the days went by villagers would arrive in the morning with their possessions tied up in bundles, take shelter, and wait for the sirens to wail. Extra trenches were dug in the village as the tide of refugees kept coming in. Totsuka was on the main road inland from the cities of Yokohama and Tokyo and the village was swelling beyond capacity. But at long last the end was definitely in sight and our only task, still, was to stay alive!

The month past into April which is the beginning of summer according to the Japanese calendar. In the country the metamorphosis was complete as the delicate pink cherry blossoms drifted down on the new green of the fields. Accompanied by the peach and plum, the petals mingled to form a fragrant carpet. Spring in the country in the northern hemisphere was a new and remarkable experience, and it cast the conflict around us temporarily aside. The different shades of green, now appearing daily, fascinated us. The lovely pale green of the chestnuts, fat spears of bamboo shooting upwards before our very eyes and the feathery willow gave the surrounding countryside a new beginning. Encircling the young trees were sprouting fields of grain and down in the hollows patchwork patterns of paddy fields. The thatched roof cottages standing amid the fields in all this spring loveliness took on a romantic look and diverted our thoughts from the wretchedness and poverty engulfing us.

The change of season brought little furry animals out of their burrows and amid the misery it was a glimpse of country life we had not expected. In this time of acute food shortage it puzzled me that the domestic animals never seemed to attempt to catch these creatures so close at hand. Was it because they were just too feeble? It was soon apparent that not everyone in this area had survived the winter. From the local cemetery new shallow graves appeared and the stench over-powered the fragrance of spring. During an air raid a few of us went over the fence to investigate the graves. Nothing edible could be found and to rue the day we came back not only thoroughly nauseous, but empty-handed as well. Anything that might have been offered to the spirits undoubtedly would have been taken by our furry neighbours.

When the full bloom of spring was really upon us it heralded more than the blossoming of cherry, plum and peach trees. There were high explosions and fragments of planes hurtling from the sky as dog fights took place. Our spirits rose daily now. Mori told us to be prepared to move as fire from incendiaries was likely. We did not want to move again. Surely no bombs would be dropped here, we couldn't be that unlucky. We were fortified with the power of ever reassuring hope these days and had no fear - perhaps foolishly - of incendiaries.

The road was filled with people carrying what they could salvage on their flight from the capital. They wore forlorn expressions carrying their babies and holding young children by the hand, a few pulled wooden carts or rode bicycles, but most of them followed, one after the other, trudging wearily on foot, with their possessions secured in bundles hanging from poles across their shoulders. These days we kept out of their way as much as possible thinking that there would be a great deal of hostility towards us, but these disheartened, retreating people showed very little animosity. My thoughts went back to that day in Rabaul when the local people fled to the bush in fear of a Japanese invasion and how the ebb and flow of the tides of war washed upon all shores.

As the raids persisted we soaked up our freedom. It was forbidden to have clothes hanging outside the buildings and no fires were allowed during raids. Cal and Maisie and any of the other girls not well stayed indoors while the rest of us watched and counted the planes. We were very amused when Kay said she had to call the Junsa if the phone rang during a raid. He of course was in his shelter.

It was a truism that we never understood the Japanese even after more than three years of their continual presence. Mori who had never tried to hide his dislike of us was now going out of his way to show us the English newspaper. The fact that a paper was still being printed in English amazed us.

The news that a member of the Diet had hauled the War Minister over the coals for suppression of information about the turning tide of the war was another surprising piece of news. This man went on to say that the people must be told the truth about their country's position and that more air raid shelters must be provided for protection against enemy bombing, which was causing destruction to many Japanese cities.

These days the Obasan and the Junsa had quite a number of visitors who came with their bundles, presumably holding all their worldly possessions. Non-officials and air raid wardens were often about and spent most of their time, when things were quiet, on the Obasan's floor deep in the ceremony accompanying the drinking of *O-cha*. These cups of hot green tea were needed now, more than ever, to give them spiritual succour.

'Taiwan finished now,' Mori revealed to us towards the end of May.

Taiwan! It was rumoured, at Vunapope, that Taiwan was to be the destination of the men who were taken from Rabaul on the *Montevideo Maru*, so there was tremendous interest in Mori's information. A good number of civilians shipped away were known to our group of Administration nurses. Sadly, among many personal friends were, also, the son and son-in-law of Mrs Bignell. Her son-in-law was a school-teacher from Kavieng; his wife had left New Guinea to have their first baby in Australia a short time before the women were evacuated, needless to say Mrs Bignell had no news of her daughter or of her expected grandchild. Missionary colleagues of the Methodist nurses, all good friends in that missionary family, were also among the civilians on the *Montevideo Maru*. Mary did not know where her husband Tom might be, she had received no information from Father Barrow or the officers who travelled with us to this so-called *paradise*. Tom Goss was not on the ship; yet where was he? For me there was Noel, always in my thoughts, thoughts of a future together, an uncertain future. Aware of the uncertainty, I would not allow myself to be obsessed by it. For Joyce it was the same, with Bill on the other side of the world fighting for his country. We had no crystal ball portraying our destiny, we had only faith in *Ashita*. Not now, tomorrow - tomorrow holds the key!

Spirits and hopes were high but gave us little true warmth; a cold wind had lain siege to the area and comfort came only from the belief that salvation was near. The weather had been fairly predictable in Japan, changing with the seasons, yet now, instead of the days getting progressively warmer, they were growing colder. The wind was constantly blowing and stripped the last struggling blossoms from the cherry trees. Our new corn and tomato plants were flattened. Mori swore that this wind was a good omen. How could it be a good omen?

'It will blow the invaders from our shores; it is God's Wind.'

He told us that he was referring to what had become a legend in Japan. In the 13th century a powerful typhoon swept Kublai Khan's mighty armada from the sacred shores of these islands and destroyed the fleet. The threatened invasion of the Mongols, thus thwarted, was never to return. The Japanese named the typhoon *Kami Kaze* (Divine Wind), believing it had been sent by the Gods to save them. Mori told us that a typhoon was a force more formidable than any mortal enemy. As air raids once more intensified, this wind of the present day, by whatever name, did not have the legendary impact.

We learnt from Mori, also, on this informative day, of a deadly attack weapon exclusive to the Japanese, the *Kamikaze* or Divine Wind Special Attack Force. Mori spoke with consummate reverence about self-sacrificing Japanese pilots, who savagely attacked the enemy and by their deeds were immortalised as Gods. A suicide mission! How could we believe the truth or even the significance of this unthinkable tactic?[4]

The Japanese acknowledged that Tokyo and Yokohama were now in ruins so we reasoned that our liberation would be only a matter of weeks, perhaps two at the most.

On July the 3rd a European man suddenly appeared in our midst. He was a representative of the International Red Cross and, as always, Tally from the Foreign Office was present, but on this occasion an official from the Japanese Red Cross joined them. Whether the European representative was as tall and handsome as we all thought at the time was debatable, we hadn't seen one of our own breed in a long while! Nevertheless, it was a wonderful surprise especially for me as that day was my birthday.

This representative of the Red Cross was very businesslike. We were absolutely astounded to learn that he had received no previous information that we were confined in Japan and had only been given permission to visit us a week ago. We were further astounded when he said that no official news of our transportation to Japan was received by the proper source, so that news could reach our relatives. It seemed we were, in effect, misplaced - lost in Japan. Why? Why were the authorities, looking after Prisoners of War, not told of our confinement here?

Inquiries were made by him, about everything concerning us, from food to clothing and even toilet requirements. It was his turn to be shocked when we told him of our lack of warm clothing and bedding during three Japanese winters. He was not in a position to give out any war news, but would see about sending us newspapers. After swarming all over him, the poor man must have been relieved to escape the nest of hornets he had discovered. He assured us that the proper authorities would be immediately informed of our whereabouts, and that he would call again at the end of the month.

The Japanese officials clung to the Red Cross representatives like blood-sucking leeches when the brief visits were allowed. We knew from past experience that in this country they had limited liberty, as to what they could do or say, so it was with some gratification that we noticed Tally looking considerably deflated on this occasion.

Interest in our welfare gave such a boost to our morale; it was the best sign we could have been given as to how serious the war situation had become for the Japs. Since we had received some Red Cross parcels during our confinement we found it hard to believe that the officials had not informed Australian authorities of our whereabouts. A few days later a group of labourers arrived to dig air raid trenches. A bit late was the general opinion. It was the middle of our fourth year in captivity and at long last we all knew for certain, "they will be here soon".

In view of all this optimism, I can only say that it must have been just plain habit that I was manuring my garden patch this day when Lik appeared.

'Drop that you're not going to reap that crop.'

She was nearly incoherent when she told me that Mori had just advised Kay that there was a peace conference soon to take place. I did as she advised and dropped it and never again turned the soil of Japan.

That night bits and pieces that had been hoarded for years were dragged out in a pseudo celebration of our anticipation of peace; we were confident events would escalate quickly and victory would be ours. Long idle lipsticks which were rather dried out were used sparingly. We would be needing them when the boys dropped in! Our appearance left a lot to be desired yet it was a sign of our elatedness that we could imagine mere lipstick would improve our looks.

White Cross ships could come and go we had no want for them; the war was about to end and we would be free at last. *Ashita* was very near.

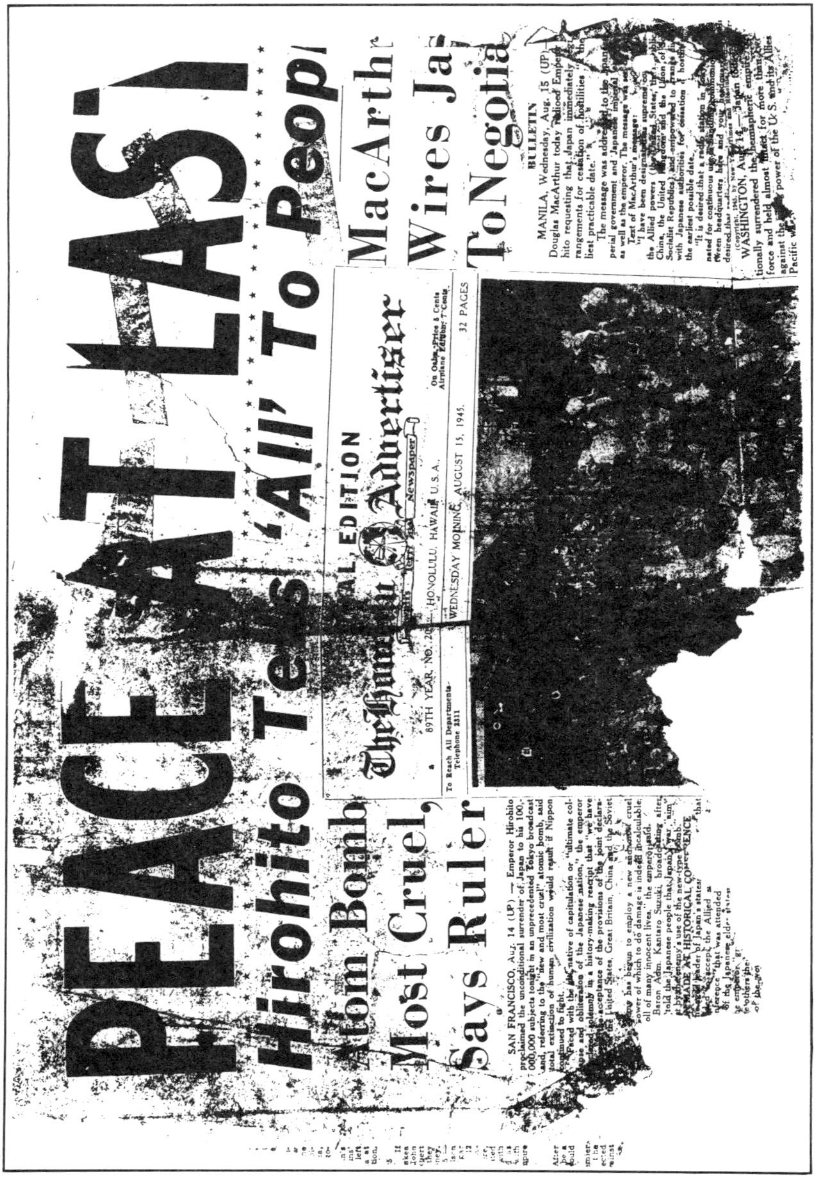

PEACE AT LAST!

Hirohito Tells 'All' To People

The Honolulu Advertiser

FINAL EDITION

89TH YEAR, NO. 20... HONOLULU, HAWAII, U.S.A. WEDNESDAY MORNING, AUGUST 15, 1945. 32 PAGES

To Reach All Departments Telephone 2311

On Oahu: Price 5 Cents. Airplane Edition: 7 Cents

Atom Bomb Most Cruel, Says Ruler

SAN FRANCISCO, Aug. 14 (UP) — Emperor Hirohito proclaimed the unconditional surrender of Japan to his 100,000,000 subjects tonight in an unprecedented Tokyo broadcast and, referring to the "new and most cruel" atomic bomb, said total extinction of human civilization would result if Nippon continued to fight.

MacArthur Wires Japan To Negotiate

BULLETIN

MANILA, Wednesday, Aug. 15 (UP) — Douglas MacArthur today radioed Emperor Hirohito requesting that Japan immediately ... arrangements for cessation of hostilities ... earliest practicable date.

WASHINGTON, Aug. 14 — Japan ... unconditionally surrendered the hemisphere ... force and held almost intact for more than ... against the ... power of the U.S. and its Allies ... Pacific ...

The Honolulu Advertiser - 15th August 1945

10

PEACE

There was rejuvenation among us. Laughter rang out. There was none of the usual, almost obligatory dissent, when proposals of dubious nature or otherwise were put forward, no hint of argument over the airing of whimsical ideas. Light-heartedness was in the air that had never been upon us before. Whether our attitude was due to the optimistic outlook of the war or a deterioration of brain cells, or maybe a combination of both, we weren't prepared to say, but it caused our happy little group to become very fanciful.

One of the missionary girls suggested that if all the Japs were as addicted to cigarettes as the Obasan was our problems would have been over long ago. The Americans could have dropped millions of tons of tobacco instead of bombs and ended the war in a matter of days. This would have spared lives, to say nothing of money, and furthermore would have made all the people happy, except perhaps the *big military men*. Another frivolous idea was prompted when constant day and night bombing resumed. In the hapless event of one of our airmen being brought down in this area, we would smuggle him, somehow, into the ceiling and use the last of our cigarettes to get food for him.

On July the 7th Mori told us that the Imperial suburb of Tokyo had been bombed. This was disturbing news, especially at this stage, and fears about repercussions were renewed. Thankfully, a further report stated that there had been no casualties. Our happy mood continued and as July came to an end we heard more mutterings about the anxiously awaited peace conference. What a most wonderful month this had been.

Strangely the Japs did not seem to care anymore that we had access to newspapers. Mori always left his paper where he knew we would see it and there were times when he actually handed it to Kay when he was finished with it. It seemed that he was now taking a fatalist view of the war, being enlightened enough to know that defeat for his country was imminent.

We read a statement in the *Nippon Times* expressing the view that the marshy land in the south was not suitable for paratroops to land. A further article made reference to a sacred feudal castle, north of Tokyo, that had kept the enemy at bay some two thousand years ago and would, somehow, come to the aid of this stricken country now in 1945.

Maps in the newspapers showed Sagami Bay and the Chiba Peninsula as likely invasion points for seaborne troops, while the airforce would encircle Tokyo. The newspaper, that a short time ago was being castigated by the Government for not telling the people the truth, was now giving out dire warnings; invasion by ground troops was imminent.

"Every man, woman and child must be prepared to take up arms and fight to the death". Another quote stated "Japanese forces are awaiting the decisive moment to smash the enemy beyond his ability to recover".

These articles in the paper gave us a strong, yet conflicting opinion that there was an influential element of power in Japan that would never give in and we wondered if that faction could stand in the way of peace. On these premises kitchen knives were sharpened with zeal and, ominously, new swords had been issued to the Junsa. The soldiers from the nearby barracks were no longer seen in the vicinity and school children stamped and drilled in their place.

Since the announcement of Peace talks the police force had been increased around this area but little notice was taken of us as we wandered further afield revelling in our new found freedom. The Junsa, who still lived on the premises, warned us daily of possible antagonism from the local people.

No longer confined, it was difficult to believe that we were still in Japan as we walked in the sunshine through the pines and cedars and beautiful chestnut trees. Our feet gave in, after about an hour of walking on them, but in spite of the handicap we appreciated for the first time the real beauty of the countryside. Not far away, however, the scene portrayed a different story - a story of struggle.

As far as the eye could see all the land was under cultivation. Before the war an estimated fifty percent of the people were engaged in agriculture and the land they tilled was at most two acres per family with every inch of soil under production. In this patterned carpet of fields there was no question that the Japanese should not be considered "the world's best gardeners"; they had no choice in a grossly overpopulated land!

As we slowly retraced our steps, I thought of those young soldiers stripping the gardens of fruit and vegetables at Vunapope and realised it was little wonder when they came from a country like this. Little wonder too, that some of them ran away into the jungle when ordered on board ship to fight for the Emperor in the Pacific.

During these last two weeks we received no further confirmation of the proposed peace and the tension at Totsuka was becoming positively electric. Reliable news in the papers was rare and our comments on the progress, or otherwise, of the war and peace negotiations tended to invite disquiet; we once again became divided into optimists and pessimists. And even I had to admit that information given us by the Junsa was as confusing as it was varied.

We were told that on 6th August one bomb, dropped on Hiroshima, had killed seventy thousand people and caused unbelievable devastation! We naturally said that such a thing was impossible and the old boy was losing his mind. Yet, a few days later the Obasan told us that a 'big' bomb had been dropped on Nagasaki and that our *danna-sans* (masters) would be coming soon.

We could not understand what all this talk about bombs, no matter how big, being dropped on far-away cities had to do with our situation. The pessimists said we had waited too long and talk of peace was all nonsense. Continual bombing for two days came once again in the middle of August and after the disastrous fires over Tokyo and the eastern seaboard these last few months we wondered what could possibly be left to destroy.

The very next morning, the 14th August, a great gathering of Japanese assembled at the Obasan's house. Loud speakers had been erected and police, field workers and school children prostrated themselves in and around her house and began praying. We stayed indoors and watched with great interest from our secret viewing spot as the ancient wireless whistled and crackled the strains of the Japanese national anthem.

The most dramatic and wonderful announcement of our lives followed, when the revered Son of Heaven, Emperor Hirohito himself, broadcast a message to his people. It was the first time his sacred voice had been heard on radio! He told his loyal seventy-five million subjects that their conflict was over. The Emperor talked of a most cruel bomb and that Japan must capitulate or be faced with ultimate collapse and the obliteration of the Japanese nation.

We only partially understood the speech but we did know it meant the days of aggression and savagery were over. Copies of the *Honolulu Advertiser*, Hawaii's territorial newspaper dated 15th August 1945 (Wednesday morning's edition) were dropped over Japan and we knew for certain that it really was PEACE AT LAST. We read with gusto those words which were three inches high! An inch-high sub-heading, "Hirohito Tells 'All' To People", described the speech as a confusing Japanese chat.

It was a very forlorn group who walked away from the Obasan's house after the Emperor's speech; many of the women were crying. The Obasan emerged unruffled and we knew that it would not be long before she would be making plans for a future in which she would remain a winner. Some of us thought she had already done so.

Early in the evening Mori sent for Kay and told her officially of the capitulation. Kay said that he too, seemed quite calm and resigned. Had the terms been rejected, Mori informed Kay, Allied paratroops were prepared for a landing.

That night, for the first time in years, we could really celebrate with millions around the world. Joyce, Lik and I opened our last tin of Bully we had been saving for just this day - we were counted among the optimists. Of course the pessimists celebrated too - we all celebrated together - but they still declared that they would not be totally convinced of victory until they actually set eyes on a Yank coming up the village path! Though the optimists needed no convincing, the idea of Americans coming up the village path to free us appealed tremendously. The contents of a packet of Old Gold cigarettes, which had been kept for a rainy day on the trading market, were greatly appreciated by the smokers. They could puff away with a clear conscience since our days of bartering were over.

Reconnaissance planes flew over on the 16th and 17th August and were fired upon by the ack-ack. Apparently not all the Japanese had accepted the cease-fire, fortunately there were no casualties.

Following the official announcement of surrender, when the initial shock had visibly lessoned, the people of Totsuka - mostly women - waylaid us at every opportunity. They were not seeking gifts or food just intercession for their lives; they seemed to be terrified of the Americans. They clustered around us calling us *okii tomadachi* (great friends, meaning - good friends) and begged us to ask the Americans not to cut their throats. Propaganda had really worked with these poor peasants!

The Obasan, alone, among the women of this area weathered the defeat of her country with her usual sangfroid; no doubt she realised she'd backed a winning horse when she kept us alive with her deals. She wore her 'Australian map' belt on the outside of her trousers. No one would be concerned now as to how she came by this gift from the enemy and very soon the Americans would be around loaded with cigarettes.

A few days after the peace broadcast Mori said a thousand *yen* would be spent on food for the internees in the camps. He did not give any details as to what department or society would be supplying this money. We had no idea of the buying power of Japanese currency and waited for the outcome without too much expectation.

It was not long before a sight we never thought we'd see in Japan appeared before us. On the 20th August a huge side of beef was delivered, along with tins of milk, salmon, butter and sugar and bottles of beer, the last thing we would have expected. Having been accustomed to only a small bowl of rice each day, unless our bargaining brought forth a few spuds, we could scarcely believe it possible that this amount of food had suddenly become available. Had Aladdin's magic lamp been found in Japan?

No more illicit cooking in tins for us. We were allowed to use the *hibachi* in the kitchen and it was no trouble to scrounge enough bamboo and such like, for stoking the fire. After eating practically day and night for a few days we could at last turn our minds to other things. However, it was not long before we were thinking of our stomachs once more. We all had acute indigestion and, ironically, there was no cure for it but to cut down on eating!

In an endeavour to control the desire to eat we walked further afield. We saw soldiers marching up to the barracks near the village to lay down their arms. Women and children watched silently, though many were crying with emotion as the young soldiers walked rigidly away without a sideward glance.

'We must pray that they are not going to commit *harakiri*,' one of the younger Missionary nurses said as we walked away. 'It's supposed to be an honourable deed for a defeated Japanese soldier.' She seemed to be talking to herself, as no one made any comment.

Since coming to Totsuka personal contact with these poor peasants had given us some insight into their burdensome lives; normally they had very little and now they had nothing at all. What humble pride they might have had seemed to be gone too. They were dispirited and we found ourselves looking on them with pity. After all we had been there not so long ago and though we had never abandoned hope of salvation we understood something of their uncertainty for the future.

In spite of the Junsa's warning, that these country people might show hostility towards us, we were often greeted with *O-hayo* (good morning) when we passed in the narrow lanes in the early morning. Having come to know that no European could ever understand the Japanese mind, or how the people were likely to react, this general politeness had little meaning. Realising the hardship and debasement that Japanese peasants took for granted, we were confident that an American/Australian occupation of their country, following the war, would be to their eventual benefit.

On 22nd August 1945, three years and seven months since the invasion of New Guinea, planes flew over to see to the disarmament of Japan. The next day in brilliant sunshine we stood spellbound while the air buzzed with the roar of engines. The skies were filled with planes with beautiful stars on their wings - no piercing red orbs now. They circled above like mighty eagles protecting the nest.

Late in the afternoon of this simply marvellous day the area around Totsuka was caught in the tail end of a typhoon. Saturated now in the euphoria of the wonderful happenings of the last few days we scarcely gave the results of this intruder a thought. The fierce winds toppled trees and flattened houses. The pouring rain made rivers in the mounds of soil where our sweet potatoes had battled for survival, and the trenches filled with water, but we didn't give a damn![1]

News of events came so frequently we had difficulty assimilating all the information. We were in a constant state of elatedness and to add to our joy we were finally allowed to write a short letter home! Mori told us that an advance fleet of naval vessels was expected on 26th of the month and these were to be followed by the remainder of the fleet on the 28th.

Mori said that a small bunch of Americans were to be billeted at the Bund Hotel. True or false we laughed anyway.

'Poor Mrs Saito' we chorused, 'accommodating the invaders. They would certainly need to be fed well, this time she will really have to find God in her heart.'

Of course the Americans would bring their own food and plenty of it and they would find a different Mrs Saito from the one we knew. The humiliation of stealing the rather unsavoury, raw vegetables from her store would not be an issue.

There were no local buses on the highway as they had been confiscated for use by the Americans. This was wonderful news that they were at least around the countryside. During the brief interval, since the peace declaration and the landing of the Americans, we did little else but eat and those of us who suffered only from malnutrition and general weakness gained strength daily.

Although the *geta* had been our sole footwear for a long time now, we found it a cumbersome accessory over the rough areas we were traversing these days. I was amazed at the variety of *geta* worn by the villagers. Some were on raised platforms at least three inches high and Mori told me that they were all made from a very special wood. Nevertheless, I had fond memories of my shoes traded for potatoes with the Obasan's brother and began to think up ways of having the bargain reversed. But it was not to be. When I did see him again he was wearing the shoes, or rather, shuffling around in them; he had cut away the heel section. The *geta* was more his line of footwear after all.

Events almost too impossible to clearly comprehend followed each other in rapid succession that our minds were in happy turmoil day and night. On the 24th August we were up at dawn, after an almost sleepless night, and waited expectantly for food to "drop from the sky". The Junsa produced a large khaki canvas, with P.O.W. appliqued in white, which was supplied by the Red Cross. After spreading it across the pumpkin patch we climbed onto the roof of our building to keep a lookout. Lovely little planes with Food Supplies painted across their tails flew around. We waved and screamed hysterically, but after sitting on the roof for some hours there was nothing forthcoming so we reluctantly climbed down. We decided that this must have been a reconnaissance exercise to sight our position, and the positions of the many other camps as well.

Later that afternoon a great hue and cry went up as one lone plane flew over and a drum was dropped some distance away in the field. We, of course, rushed to the spot only to find a fine mess of stew and fruit salad where the drum had dropped without a parachute. This was not the catastrophe it would have been a few months earlier and we cheerfully salvaged what we could from the wreckage.

With each day something exhilarating happened and we became more and more overjoyed.

'Look what's coming down over there.'

Shrieks from Whytie and Lik sent us barefoot across the field. Drifting down gracefully were parachutes of every colour imaginable, from pale blues to purples, orange reds and whites. They looked like bunches of beautiful mushrooms floating from heaven that could have come straight out of a Walt Disney fantasy. But, of course, they contained more items of food.

An old Irish priest arrived in our midst another day, looking exhausted after walking a long way. The day was unusually hot for August and it gave us great pleasure to be able to offer him real tea and biscuits, to say nothing of the pleasure it gave having someone so keen to listen to us for the first time in so long. Cal was very sick now, gravely ill, although the nourishing food had revived her a little. Cal was a devout Catholic and the Father immediately went in to see her; he stayed with her for a while and gave her the last rites. Help was on the way and we hoped she could hold on.

The Father had only yesterday heard of us when he visited the Swiss Legation in Tokyo. He had come to Japan as a missionary thirty years earlier and when the war started missionaries and neutrals of various countries had not actually been interned, but had to remain within certain boundaries and report regularly to the authorities.

He came from a Mission at Fukishima north of Tokyo and told us that he hadn't had much opportunity to speak English as most of the other internees were of foreign nationality. Whole families were confined there and quite a few were brought to Japan after the capture of their ship by a German raider in the Indian Ocean, quite early in the war. Their ship, the *Nankin*, was taken by the raider after abandonment off the coast of Western Australia and passengers and crew were picked up and transferred to a German prison ship and eventually transported to Japan. The Father believed the crew of this merchant ship, which included Australian Naval ratings to man its defensive guns, were imprisoned elsewhere in Japan. We were beginning to hear already of fellow prisoners of war! We assured him we could listen indefinitely to an English voice giving us so much interesting news and hoped he would stay as long as possible.

It absolutely astonished us to hear that New Britain had not been retaken. The people there still in captivity? This was quite distressing news as we had assumed that Rabaul would have been liberated when the Americans launched their counter-offensive in the Pacific. The war was over and we found it hard to believe that so many Japanese were in Rabaul and still in control. The Father received his information when a Japanese officer in Rabaul had relayed it by letter to his wife, who was a member of the Father's diocese. From the middle of 1943 as the Americans began to win back the Pacific the Japs in Rabaul were in little communication with Japan and became seriously dependant on their own resources. It was reported that Japanese on some of the islands were so desperately short of food they had resorted to cannibalism!

We now had confirmation that the war in Europe had been over since May and that Hitler and Mussolini were dead. His information that the people were on the verge of starvation as there was very little food in Japan, we already knew. He told us that President Rooseveldt had died in April and our own Prime Minister, John Curtin, only weeks ago, just before the final victory. It was sad to think that these two leaders, who had strived so hard for their countries, could not share the triumph.

He told us of the bombs dropped on Hiroshima and Nagasaki that had never been used against the enemy before and that the destruction really was as terrible as we had heard. When the Japanese refused to accept the surrender terms offered, the Allies were left no option but to employ these newly developed atom bombs to put an end to the war. His information was that all prisoners of war were to be immediately executed if the Allies had landed on Japanese soil. We were certainly pleased we had not known of this earlier, although there had been rumours to that effect. He also told us the surprising news of Russia's entry into war with Japan. Japan was devastated when Russia invaded Manchuria, as late as August the 8th, and defeat was inevitable. The Japs had taken Manchuria from Russia in 1931 when Japan began her new policy of expansion.

We told the Father that we had heard so many rumours about the war we could never tell fact from fiction and, as he replied, he smiled for the first time.

'After thirty years I still do not know how the Japanese think and I do not believe all they say, either.'

When it was time for the old priest to leave he graciously refused the offer of food from our plentiful supply.

'Thank you, but all will be well now that the Americans have come.' We certainly agreed with that.

I suppose it must be said that the 30th August was just about the most exciting day of our lives. Two of the girls on patrol duty after lunch sighted a General Headquarters staff car - perhaps it was General MacArthur himself - followed by several vehicles speeding towards Yokohama from the direction of Atsugi Aerodrome. Atsugi, we learned recently, was not very far from here to the south west, and this explained why there had been so much aircraft activity around Totsuka. The girls waved and yelled frantically at the Americans, but without apparent recognition. They raced all the way back to give us the news and for the rest of the day we haunted the roadway. Late in the afternoon we were rewarded when several truck-loads of soldiers swept by on their way to Yokohama. One of the lads, sitting in a rather precarious position, nearly fell off the truck when we appeared near the hedge. The convoy did not stop, but we knew they had seen us, and we had seen them, and it would not be long now.

Next day I was sitting on my mat thinking pleasant thoughts when my visions of the future were abruptly interrupted by a frightful shrieking and stampeding. In the corridor pinned to the wall was a very tall American officer and a smaller edition beside him was a private receiving similar treatment as more of the nurses converged on the scene. When these two were able to make themselves heard they introduced themselves as Major Meanley of the 11th Airborne Division and his driver. They said they had been waylaid on the highway in the pouring rain by two girls - Whytie and Lik - "dragged out of our vehicle and brought up to this camp". Kay slipped away to tell Cal the wonderful news that the Yanks had arrived and to prepare her for the sight.

These men were just marvellous and within half an hour they had produced a doctor. The poor man had just arrived by plane and had not yet had time for breakfast or a shave, he told us later. He spoke to Cal and let us know that he would arrange for her to be placed on a hospital ship immediately.

Major Meanley was anxious to know our opinion of the Japs. He told us that when the motorcade escorted General MacArthur into

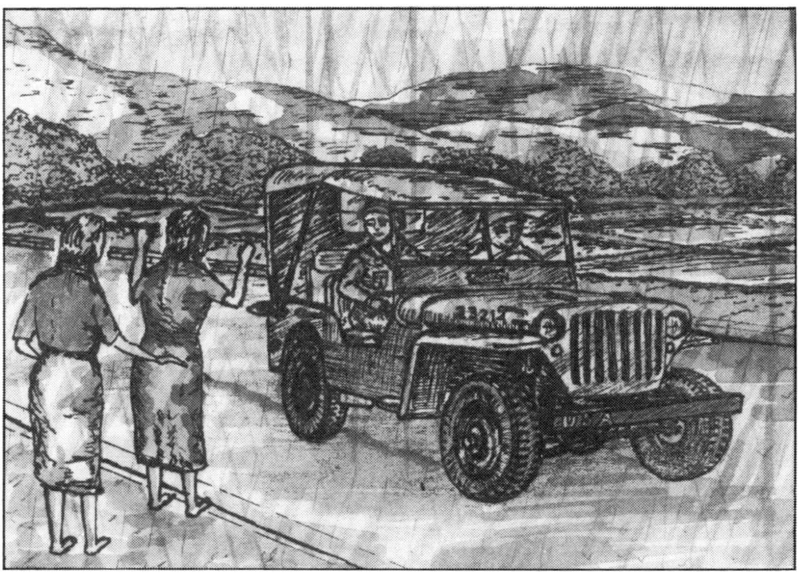

Waylaid on the highway by Whytie and Lik

Yokohama the roads were lined at intervals with Japanese soldiers carrying rifles. On approach of the American vehicles the soldiers turned away from the road and held their rifles at present arms. The Americans were not able to learn why this was done even after two reasons were put forward. The first, which was preferred, was that this honour was to protect them from ambush; the second, because of their country's dishonour in defeat, was to show contempt for the victors. From our experience we could be of no assistance as we had always found the Japs to be enigmatic.

When we reluctantly had to part with our captives we escorted them to the highway; it was raining all the time but we really didn't notice it. The Major told us, laughingly, that this had been the hottest battle he had been in for a long time and his driver lapping up the attention seemed to be thoroughly enjoying himself.

'Boy, could I take a lot more of this,' he said.

Their vehicle, we were told, was called a jeep and as we hadn't seen one before we gave it a kiss and as we hadn't seen men like these two in such a long time we treated them in a similar manner. They drove off telling us we'd be seeing them and more like them, *real soon*.

Our own Australian boys arrived that evening to what can only be described as a warm welcome. It was truly remarkable how one reacts to the sound of army boots - our Army boots - they made the most musical sound in the whole world! The boys wound their way through debris that now almost completely obstructed the corridor. There were food boxes around, items of clothing being aired, swags in readiness and remains of 'rubbish' saved over our years of confinement. After hoarding for so long we found it almost impossible to part with anything. The Aussie boys demonstrated such wonderful patience as they tried to extract information from us and particulars, regarding family matters, in the dim light provided by a piece of rag in a saucer of butter. Oh! What a waste this was! The electric power had been disrupted by a parachute falling on the lines when we were bombarded with food a few days ago.

All we wanted to do was talk to them, and attempt to find out the news of the past years in a few hours. We asked them everything from musicals to songs now popular, the Royal family, what was happening in Australia now and of course about New Guinea. They seemed to have no information about New Guinea and knew nothing of the men taken away in the *Montevideo Maru*. Japan was crowded with so many prisoners of war whose camps had not been located yet and the Australians had no idea of the numbers being held. We told them everything Ducky had passed on to us about his internment and the conditions he had encountered before coming to the Club in 1943. We had also given this information to the Americans earlier.

During these final days the Obasan had faded into the background, though she was never far away. When the Australians came to see about our passports and numerous other particulars, the Obasan quietly appeared among us and sat-in on this session. The men did not take kindly to this intrusion until we explained our bargaining deals with her and they softened a little; we added that she did not understand English. We didn't explain that while this was strictly true, she never once had any trouble understanding us!

For a while now the Obasan had been sending her children to help us, by cleaning our rooms and gathering bamboo and pieces of wood for our now ever-burning stove. Had old Fuji seen us in action in his kitchen I am sure he would have suffered a stroke. He had plagued our lives since the beginning and when he left after the incendiary bombing of Tokyo we never saw him again.

Two young Americans, Bernie and Sam, were brought to us by an American officer who handed them over for safe keeping; they too had been prisoners in Japan.

'They have nowhere else to go and we know you girls will take good care of them.' Before he left, this officer asked if we needed anything. We replied that we had everything except bread which we had not seen for a long time.

'You will have it right here today,' he said cheerfully as he saluted us and left.

At first it was impossible to get any information from either of these two Americans, they simply never stopped eating! But eating was all we had been doing for the past week also.

Eventually after a hearty meal Bernie and Sam, who were captured at Corregidor in 1942, told us a little of their story as prisoners of war over the last few years. When put on board a ship bound for Taiwan they were harassed by allied submarines and chased about the ocean before reaching Hong Kong. Seven hundred were battened down in the hold where there was barely sitting room and conditions were so bad that close to a hundred men died and many lost their minds. At Hong Kong they were allowed on deck for only fifteen minutes. The ship finally set out for Taiwan and when they arrived not one man could walk. The survivors were brought to Japan where they were imprisoned in Kobe for the duration of the war.

When peace was declared these two broke out of the Kobe camp and hitched their way to Yokohama where they were picked up by the 11th Airborne Division. After listening to this tragic story we were tongue-tied and all thinking of our men on the *Montevideo Maru*. We knew the great number crammed on board that ship; had they been forced to endure this inhuman suffering?

Our pensive mood changed once again to joy when an American vehicle arrived and the driver delivered a sack of bread, which was especially baked for us and just flown in from Okinawa. Was it not surprising we thought the Yanks were wonderful?

The Australians who had been taking down our particulars said they would see us tomorrow and if the weather proves favourable we would probably be flown to Okinawa in the afternoon. What difference did one day matter after all this time?

'Ima nai, Ashita,' I said aloud in Japanese. The Obasan's frequently repeated words were ringing in my mind.

Not now, tomorrow. Whether tomorrow or the next day, tomorrow was here and nothing mattered anymore.

Another welcome visitor brought by the Australians was Captain Forrester, a Queenslander. There was scarcely any break in the conversation that night. Someone was always ready to take over after a few minutes silence to catch the breath.

Most of us were up and about early the next morning. We had talked enough over the years on the subject of what we would do when our men arrived and, now they were here, we set out to make them feel at home. The Captain said he'd "never got the coffee habit" and as we had an abundance of tea in our parcels we were happy to please him. To really give these boys a hearty breakfast we sent the Obasan to the village to scrounge for eggs.

After our meal news came through that our departure was postponed until tomorrow. We would be billeted for the night at Atsugi and fly out in the morning.

At last! We climbed on to a rickety Japanese bus at the roadside. Mori, who was still in residence, unveiled the ultimate hypocrisy by telling us to take good care of ourselves. The Obasan stood by dressed in her best *kimono*. As she called out *Sayonara* she raised her arm and we saw that she had two packets of American cigarettes tucked in her *obi*. Somehow we were relieved to know that someone was already taking care of her.

Just as had happened more than three and a half years ago the rain came down in torrents and the old bus was bogged in the mud; not for long though, there were plenty of willing helpers this day. However, Bernie was not one of them he was too busy munching on a large hunk of cheese.

Two officers of the 11th Airborne Division took us on a tour of Atsugi Airfield after our arrival. We seemed to go around in circles. The Americans told us that this huge airport was one of the finest in the world.

'Is that why you never bombed it?'

The question produced a flurry of grinning faces!

That evening we had our first taste of social life in years and after a lavish supper we finally got into bed about 1am. We had real mattresses and yards of stiff new sheeting - what a luxury - but there was no bath. This building had been recently completed and the water was not yet laid on; how like the Japs. Next morning a long remembered breakfast of bacon and eggs, hot toast melting with butter, jam and honey, coffee and orange juice and lots of fruit was laid out for us. The cooks seemed a bit embarrassed when we thanked them later. To us it was all too wonderful.

On 2nd September 1945 General MacArthur became overlord of Japan and the Emperor was now a *puppet* figure. As peace was being signed aboard the USS *Missouri* in Tokyo Bay, eighteen oddly attired and rather scruffy, but marvellously happy women climbed aboard a C-54 Skymaster. The Americans told us we were almost making an inaugural flight, as this was a brand new luxury aeroplane just in service. Cal had been taken out earlier and was being cared for aboard a hospital ship in Tokyo Bay along with many fellow prisoners of war. Tokyo Bay was filled with hundreds of ships of the Allied nations which had been at war with Japan.

We were the first group of prisoners, which included Bernie and Sam and other boys who soon made themselves known to us, to leave Japan. We flew east over Tokyo Bay, the Naval Depot, Chiba Peninsula and Oshima (Big Island) before heading south. The pilot said he would have liked to have flown over Tokyo and Yokohama to show us the aftermath of the bombing, but this risk he couldn't take.

'Seeing you are all so keen to get back to Aussie.'

Half an hour later the only thing visible of Japan was the ghostlike summit of Fujiyama. As it faded into oblivion we glimpsed our last sight of that place of distasteful memories. Below us, white-capped waves revelled in a sea cleansed with freedom and ahead, clear blue skies paved the way for *tomorrow*. We had left Japan.

On arrival at Okinawa we were surprised to see ambulances standing by at the airport. We disembarked and were standing about on the tarmac when one of the pilots called out to the ambulance men.

'You won't need those buses for this bunch, unless you'd like to take them for a ride!'

11

MANILA

The next morning was the fifth anniversary of the beginning of the Second World War and we were off again. We were heading for Manila where we would be staying a few days to recuperate before our homeward bound journey. We took to the air from Okinawa in a troop carrier. The aircraft, a C-46 Commando, was not such a luxury liner as yesterday but we were flying higher. Aircraft travel was an exciting experience and, today, imaginations were stimulated as we looked down on a layer of floating clouds. The clouds took the shape of icebergs drifting through an endless sky; at other times the shapes transformed into scoops of long-forgotten ice cream. The cooler air was welcome too, after the stifling heat of yesterday, which had detracted from the glamour of padded seats and curtained port-holes.

We had to leave Marjorie Anderson behind in Okinawa as she was stricken, suddenly, with a serious bout of Malaria. There were thirty-six passengers aboard today and not as many heads drooping over paper bags as yesterday. A talkative Dutchman from Malaya had his arm in a sling.

'A bag fell out of the sky and knocked me over,' he shrugged, 'but I did not mind. We had a big feast in the camp that night, enough compensation for being the victim of a parachute drop.'

There was on board a young man who said he'd prefer to travel by ship than by plane. He had only one leg. His companions told us that he had lost his limb in the prison camp through neglect and the unhygienic conditions. We would be hearing many tragic stories of the atrocities of this war as time unfolds and of the courage welded in the hearts of men and women who were brutally treated.

'Next time I will go by sea where there is plenty of dancing and sports,' he tauntingly suggested.

'The Americans have just about thought of everything for the comfort of their passengers,' Joyce said out loud as we were invited to help ourselves to the sumptuous food laid out on a small table. We were delighted to find piles of magazines strewn about on the long wooden seats lining the sides of the cabin. There was no question of discomfort, as far as we were concerned it was sheer luxury and lots of merrymaking.

Between intervals of exchanging news, disclosing sentiments of our lives in captivity and revealing plans for the future, we read the magazines. There were great surprises in them and in the newspapers. Joyce drew my attention to a picture of Princess Elizabeth, now grown up, followed by Mr Churchill, hardly changed at all.

'Here's something that can be put straight and we won't be arguing over again,' said one of the girls. It was the date of the British Prime Minister's birthday, and I immediately thought how it seemed so unimportant that this trivial matter could have caused so much ado. There were reports of murders, suicides and other frightful topics with direct bearing on the war, and we learnt of *ethnic cleansing* that atrocious creation of Adolf Hitler's in Jewish concentration camps. How could such a philosophy be tolerated?

The most astonishing headline on the front page of the newspapers featuring articles on the Japanese Emperor was simply titled Hirohito in huge block letters. There was not one gracious, supreme, worshipful or any devout adjective preceding his name! After the last three and a half years of witnessing the esteem with which he was held, we found this surprising until we became familiar with the terms of surrender which demanded the Emperor be stripped of his Godlike status forever.

After a trip of just under five hours a group of very excited people landed at Manila. The Rabaul Sisters, as we were collectively called, were taken to the service women's compound which was surrounded by a barbed wire fence and policed day and night by armed guards. All the service women wore trousers and it took us some time to get used to this uniform. We were not convinced that the strict Matrons of the big hospitals in Australia would approve, but we had to remind ourselves that we had been lost in time and no doubt the war would have brought forth many changes.

Officially we were referred to as *recovered personnel* or simply *recovered* Prisoners of War. We said that these references made us feel like pieces of mislaid baggage even though we were well aware that we looked like mislaid vagrants of three and a half years standing.

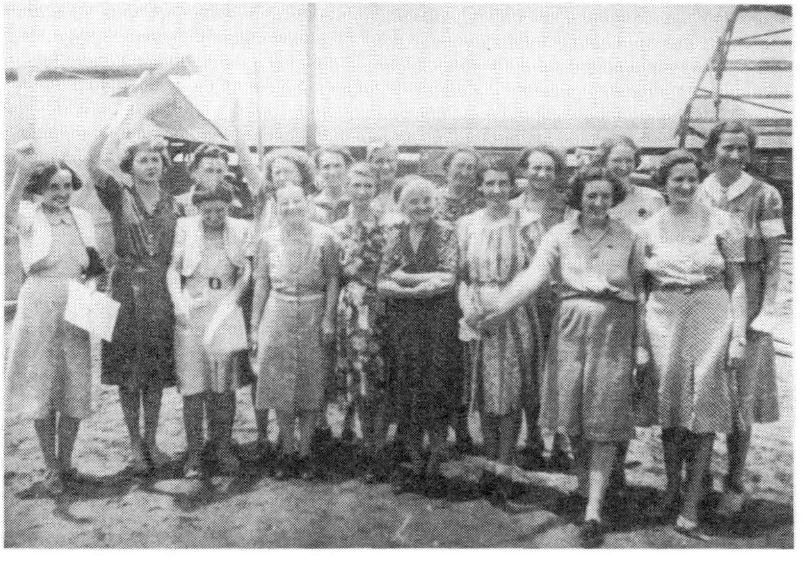

The Rabaul Nurses photographed at Manila (AWM neg.19146)

Back row L to R: Grace Kruger, Bowie (in black), Joyce McGahan, Dorothy Beale, Dora Wilson, Joyce Oldroyd-Harris, Mary Goss, Mrs Bignell, Mavis Cullen and Kay Parker.
Front row L to R: Jean McLellan, Jean Christopher, Dorothy Maye, Mrs Jones, Mavis Green, Lorna Whyte and Daisy Keast.
Sick in hospital: Eileen Callaghan and Marjorie Anderson.

The American Army, the Australian and American Red Cross and the Australian Comfort Fund provided us with every essential. We were given clothing, underwear, shoes and cosmetics, anything we wanted to drink, from coke to beer, and cigarettes for the smokers. And, as far as food was concerned, we only had to say we fancied something and it was before us. In the mess we were the first to be seated and never allowed to queue for meals, as was necessary in the large mess. We were thoroughly spoilt!

We had a quiet giggle about the way the Americans made tea in the mess. It was made in large enamel jugs, the kind that could to be found standing in a wash basin in the bedrooms of our country hotels! The jugs were not covered and the tea soon became cold. The Yanks retaliated by saying that they never did get a decent cup of coffee in Australia and then quickly added that this was really the only thing they had against the Aussies.

Our days were taken up with filling in papers and receiving medical attention and having photographs taken. Strangely, we felt the heat a great deal after the mild northern summers we had become accustomed to. In the evenings the Americans put on film shows which we ranked the best treat of all after food. After a few days rest in Manila Mrs Jones said good-bye to us. Along with Bernie and Sam she was flown home to America. Mrs Jones was an unassuming and uncomplaining woman, who had suffered a great loss and stood up to the years of hardship well. She survived the ordeal in mind and body, as well as, and in some cases better than, those half her age.

There was a marvellous surprise for us one day on being told we had a visitor waiting, someone we knew; no other than Keith Munro was standing before us. We had last seen him when he came to Namanula two days before the Jap landing and offered the alternate of escaping inland in the hope of being picked up. He told us that he had got away from the south coast along with many others at the onset of the Jap occupation. The chartered Qantas Empire Flying Boat which picked them up carried a load of men far beyond its capacity of forty. Now here he was working with the Americans. Of course we talked for hours, we had a lot to say. Keith had no knowledge of the men, many of whom were his compatriots, shipped to Japan from Rabaul. As no one had known of our own whereabouts until we were discovered and *recovered* we thought nothing of this at this early stage of locating prisoners of war. The fate of people at the Mission was not known either. The Japs had not surrendered in New Britain yet, which we already knew, and it was Keith's understanding that there were tens of thousands of them in Rabaul.

We were taken into Manila when the formalities were over and given ten pounds each donated by the Australian Government, our first real money since our last pay in Rabaul. Filipinos were riding in the streets in gaily painted carts pulled by rickshaw men. We asked a young girl if we could hire one of these and were both staggered and amused at her negative reply. They were too dangerous for us!

Few buildings had escaped the bombing and subsequent torching by the Japs as they fled; the city seemed to be just a sad mass of debris. We spoke to a few Europeans encountered and those who had come from Europe said they had never seen such devastation as here. If we were any judge we were sure that they would have said the same of Tokyo and Yokohama. Sadly, with all ruins of man's destruction so much history is destroyed and can never be replaced.

Half way between this part of Manila and our compound was the old walled city of Intramuros, the fortification built by the Spaniards in the late 16th century. The Japanese had taken their last suicidal defensive here and for six days fought to the death leaving the old city in ruins - the only building left intact was the old church. We had a lot of trouble finding a gap through the wall, but at last found ourselves inside, curiously, among the ruins of what was once an aquarium. Picking our way through the rubble of broken glass and, not surprisingly, heaps of human bones we came to the remains of tanks where some of the glass was still intact. It had obviously been a huge place in what was an underground cave where water still dripped from the roof. There was a death-like smell about the place that reminded us of the shallow graves at Totsuka.

Out in the sunlight once more we walked on to the old church of St Augustine. This church survived the destructive earthquake of 1862 and a civil uprising, which broke out in 1890 and lasted until well after the Philippines were ceded to the Americans by the Spanish, but the recent war left it badly battered. The monastery was destroyed. The priests and about two hundred others, who had taken refuge, were slaughtered by the Japanese who were determined to make a last desperate stand in Manila. Inside the church, miraculously, there was no damage at all except for some bullet holes high up in the windows. Old Spanish gilded coaches stood in the aisles of the immense interior and no one could tell us how these unusual museum pieces came to be there.

The caretaker directed us up a flight of stairs which we had to climb in a half crawling position. The passage was dark and rather eerie before we came out at the top of the bell tower and gazed over the ruins of the city. Manila was known as the Pearl of the Orient before the war. Tourists from all over the world once came to enjoy its exotic beauty, a Spanish setting in an Eastern country. After virtually slithering down the stairs we signed the visitors' book and gave a small contribution to the rebuilding fund of this piece of history.

Out of the town area there were still some beautiful homes left untouched by the war. These Spanish villas were surrounded by gaily painted walls enclosing gardens with fountains. Inside, beautiful hand-painted madonnas and cherubs looked down from the ceilings onto intricate mosaic floors and winding staircases to a mezzanine level. These lovely homes were temporarily the residences of the American occupation forces.

On our way back to the compound we turned off the highway and visited the lavish Manila Hotel, miraculously it had been untouched by bombing and was now General Headquarters. Here we were shown over the downstairs area and marvelled at the size of the dining rooms and a ballroom that looked as large as a football field. The floor was protected from the tread of Army boots by a thick canvas covering.

One afternoon we visited Las Pinas to see the San Jose Church with the only bamboo organ in the world. It was built by the local priest in 1816 and was a truly remarkable piece of work which had taken him almost ten years to perfect. While here we heard noises in the courtyard and were guided by an old priest to an upstairs window and there below was a Filipino funeral in progress. The coffin was lifted from a donkey cart and carried into the church by relatives, followed by girls looking very pretty in their lace mantillas. They were singing hymns and carrying lighted candles. After the priests had offered prayers there were more hymns while the procession moved to the churchyard burial grounds for the final rites.

We questioned the old priest about the Japanese occupation period and found him reluctant to talk about it. When we told him we had just come from Japan, and who we were, he relaxed and related the now familiar story of death, destruction and famine. There were many captured Japanese, now prisoners on this island of Luzon; others were coming down from the hills daily. It was rumoured that hostile Filipinos were 'popping them off', indiscreetly; thousands of Filipinos were slaughtered by the Japs during their final defensive. The priest told us too that of one hundred thousand Japs who had survived the fighting seventy thousand committed *harakiri*.[1] This old man said he had come from Belgium as a missionary forty years ago and since the war ended everyone had to be wary of communication with strangers, and of views expressed. In this very poor area the natives were growing hostile towards Europeans as well; many centuries of foreign ownership found the people discontent. We could detect that he felt he had revealed enough to us so we took our leave and got back to the compound without delay. We had no wish to meet with any hostile people.

Just before we left for Australia two of the officers who had travelled *de luxe* in the freighter with us to Japan came to see us. They looked many years older. Although they told us that the camp they had been interned in, Zentsuji, was a comparatively decent one, they had been close to death from malnutrition. There was more to tell, but three and a half years of ordeal could not be covered in a moment. According to their information mail for us had arrived at Zentsuji and the Japanese would not hand it over to officials from the Foreign Office. The Japs simple explanation was that our mail and bundles that arrived for the men on the *Montevideo Maru* would not be needed. In a warehouse in Yokohama mail for prisoners was discovered by the occupation forces; the letters had been stored since August 1942.

Our time was running out in Manila. There had been so much done for us during our short stay. American dentists worked on our teeth and did all they could to have us looking presentable for our arrival home, and the doctors paying attention to our health and well-being gave us last minute vaccinations. The paper work regarding *recovered personnel* was finally completed and we were cleared to go home at last.

On our second last night Keith invited us to his apartment, which was in the ruined remains of the Women's University. Joyce and I helped him cook supper and we quite enjoyed this last effort in a foreign country in the cooking line. We sipped our drinks on the balcony, minus its railing, and looked out through the blackened arches and naked framework of this once massive building. The setting sun softened the ruins and presented an unforgettable picture of the treasured city. Down below there were pools of water in the remains of the swimming baths. After a few glasses of a drink called Manila Magic we quite believed Keith when he said that sometimes in the night the mermaids down there would sing to him!

'I'm taking you girls to a nightclub,' said Keith on our last night in Manila.

Much as we wanted to go we couldn't see ourselves at a nightclub in our present attire, grateful as we were to the Red Cross and others for these clothes. We didn't need much persuasion though, when Keith suggested we just sit in a corner with a few drinks. The nightclub had an exotic island atmosphere, with grass mats on the floor and bamboo pole walls and it featured a very good string band. Filipinos, like all islanders, are very musical and we did enjoy that evening. The Filipino girls with flowers in their silken hair took our thoughts back to New Britain where the islanders were never without this symbolic floral adornment. They looked delightful in their colourful form-fitting dresses with wide airy sleeves, so elegant. We certainly did feel conspicuous; we stood out like Australian hill-billies from Steele Rudd's celebrated *Dad and Dave* series.

On our return to the compound Keith gave us letters for Heather and a few messages before we said goodbye.

'I'll be seeing you in Sydney before too long,' he said. 'And remember that day in Rabaul when I asked you all to come away with me, and you turned me down, well I'll ask you again when I come South and you'd better not turn me down this time.'

'We certainly won't Keith you can bet on that,' we said with glee.

'Oh! And you'd better not tell Heather about the mermaids!'

12

HOME AT LAST

We left the compound on the 12th September after gathering together our, by now, far more extensive belongings and saying our good-byes. We had been here over a week and we were speechless with gratitude at the kindness and generosity showered on us, nevertheless, we tried our best to thank them. We were a little surprised with the Americans' reply.

'Aw, that's all right just tell them down there that we are not as bad as they thought we were and don't believe all you might hear about us.'

No one in Manila or elsewhere had given us any cause to think there could be dissension between the Australians and the Americans and we were left quite puzzled by this remark.

'See you soon when we get home,' said the Aussie boys happily.

We were heading for Darwin which was a long ten hour hop from Manila and most of us were quiet on this trip. Thoughts that plagued our minds for so long would soon be transformed into reality. We would be going our separate ways, parting, and I wondered how long it might take to adjust to life again after our absence from it.

When the flat, dry, though water combed country of the Northern Territory appeared below no words could express the joy and at the same time relief that overwhelmed us.

This entry to Australia, via the top end, is often referred to as coming in by the back door, with Darwin Airport personifying a lack-lustre welcome. Darwin Airport was on Australian soil and the windswept, treeless country below was *home* - that was the all important thing that mattered to me, and the rest of us, after our years of isolation in Japan.

Excitement mounted as we left the plane, quite literally walking on air after the long trip. People were everywhere milling around wanting to talk to us. So grateful was Chris to be home that she recovered a stone from the airport - an Australian stone - as a memento of her safe return from *paradise*.

The hospital where we were accommodated for the night was cheerful and bright with flowers. The long low wooden buildings were cooled by the sea breeze and the nurses looked more familiar in their grey uniforms and caps, and in skirts rather than trousers. Most of us were sick as a result of the vaccinations and went to bed early. The next morning we started on the last leg of this long journey home. The sector from Darwin to Sydney would take us around twelve hours.

We had started out from Atsugi in what was a luxury aircraft, then a troop carrier from Okinawa to the Philippines; the flight home was in a B-24 bomber. Six of us had to stand in the bomb rack when taking off but afterwards we travelled in real luxury. There were mattresses laid out in the cabin, and since we were still feeling rather unwell, probably due to excitement more than the effect of our vaccinations, we were thankful to be able to sleep on this final day in the air. It was a coincidence, which I thought significantly appropriate, that we were being delivered home from imprisonment in an aircraft called a Liberator!

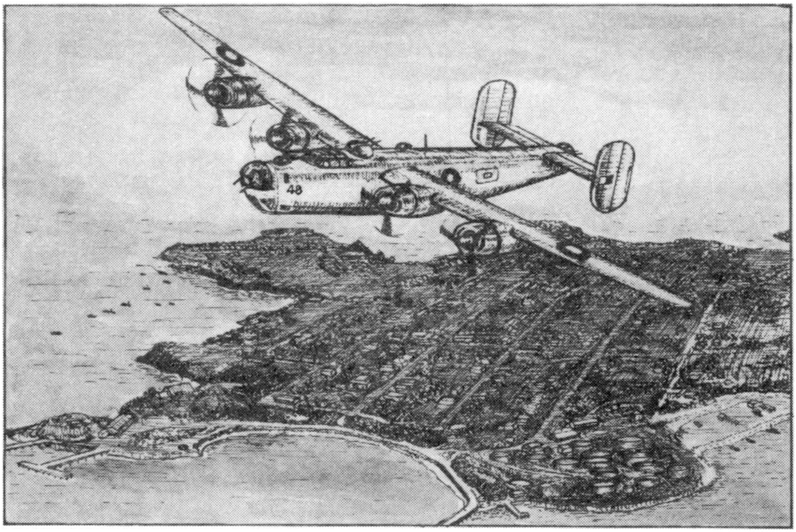

Our Liberator over Darwin

No one could have prepared us for the welcome at Mascot. Being one of the six making ballast in the bomb rack I was the first to drop out. Flashlights blinded me as photographs were taken by the press and the crowd of friends and relatives who swarmed forward. How well dressed and glamorous the women looked, they all seemed to be decked in furs and flowers, but the flowers were for us. Surrounded by emotionally happy relatives we naturally became separated from one another. My mother had not arrived in Sydney yet and an unexplained feeling overcame me. All of a sudden I felt quite dumb and was very conscious of my khaki socks and shoes, a bit too large for me, nevertheless I was thankful I didn't have to arrive home barefooted.

Our arrival was all so unreal it was almost as if fading out of a dream, however, our senses were jolted when our old friend Taffy appeared on the scene. We had not known if Taffy had escaped from Madang where she was the lone Administration nurse when the Japs came. She told us that, in company with two well known mining pioneers of the mainland and about thirty other men, she trekked five hundred miles through the jungle and over the mountains until the party reached the safety of Mount Hagen. When word finally reached Australia in May the party had grown to eighty and Taffy did a wonderful job looking after the sick. They were eventually rescued from Mount Hagen by two Qantas DH86 aircraft, in what was a magnificent feat in that mountainous area and at that early stage of the war. Ironically, later on in Sydney when she applied to join the Army she was turned down because she had flat feet!

We had no trouble recognising one another's relatives, they had all been described in minute detail over the years. After the initial impact of reunion had settled down relatives were brought forward to be introduced and they were greeted with: 'Oh! I know who you are, favourite Aunt Mary.' And 'You are Jimmie, the young brother who is always in trouble!' And from a distance came 'I bet that glamorous lass over there is *Myrna Loy*, Oldroyd's sister.'

We couldn't identify any boyfriends, many were still in the services and others were 'just missing', but we were to find out about them later. After lots of discussions, tears of joy and the like we were sorted out and driven to various destinations. The Army girls and Missionary nurses were taken to their headquarters, whilst Mrs Bignell and a few others were taken off by relatives who lived in Sydney. Those of us not from New South Wales, who were mostly Queenslanders, were booked into a hotel to await the arrival of kin.

Within the next few days various members of our families

arrived and stayed with us at the hotel. Shopping was more difficult than we thought it would be, getting used to not only having money to spend, but trying to make up our minds what to buy. There was just too much of everything! Clothes were rationed, but we were given extra coupons for these and for food also. This latter item was one thing we didn't have any trouble spending money on. Our hotel provided only bed and breakfast and we delighted in eating out; after a few days we knew every cafe and restaurant in the vicinity.

At last Joyce was reunited with Bill. Joyce's Bill was the first man in our lives to join us on our return. He served with the AIF in the Middle East and was among the troops called back to fight in the New Guinea campaign. After the fall of Rabaul Bill had written, from the Middle East, to the Australian Authorities requesting news of Joyce and he was forwarded a reply stating details of her capture and imprisonment in Vunapope. Along with many letters, including my own, Joyce's letter from Vunapope, sent in that questionable mail delivery of the Japs in April 1942, had reached its destination of Port Moresby after all. Bill was still in the Army on our return and was granted leave in Sydney to greet Joyce; his strong support gave us self-assurance when it was most needed.

We were the first prisoners to arrive home from the war and were accorded such acclaim as to be almost heroic. As the mopping-up continued, stories began to unfold of the truly atrocious treatment of other nurses in captivity, in the islands of Indonesia. I knew how fortunate we were to have been sent to Japan; we were the only group of nurses, prisoners of war, in the Land of the Rising Sun.

We were to discover that not all people were moved by the tribulation of war. There was a detachment among the populace, almost as if 'life as normal' had never been interrupted. Sometimes, I think startled shopkeepers took us for a group of bush-whackers let loose in the city for the first time, so exhilarated were we. There was the day in Pitt Street when one of the girls asked me for a loan and I just stopped where I was and hauled out a roll of notes. It was about a hundred pounds and I was immediately pounced on by my mother and told that ten pound notes were not the same as *yen* and that I was in danger of losing them in such a public place.

At the jewellers I was told that you couldn't buy ear rings for pierced ears because gold, which was not available, was the only metal suitable to be put through the ears. This gave us a good laugh as most of us used wires and pins in our ears at Totsuka, and Lik had two very long safety pins that came down almost to her shoulders. I must admit though that our ears did turn septic after a while!

Another day Joyce and I paid a visit to the famous King's Cross, a *must* for anyone visiting Sydney. A derelict old woman in a battered hat, shapeless dress and sandshoes was standing by when Joyce started to cough. She tapped Joyce on the shoulder and advised her to lie on her side on a hard floor and that would soon fix her up.

'You won't be able to sleep too well though dearie, you don't look like you could stand up to too much hardship.' I am sure she thought we were quite rude when we began to giggle.

As more and more prisoners of war returned to Australia we heard of the inhumanity of such places as the Burma Railway, where Lik lost one of her brothers among the three thousand prisoners who died horrific deaths, and of Changi Prison camp in Singapore, where three and a half years of atrocities haunt its walls. In the scattered island camps and, almost unbelievably as far as we were concerned, many of the prison camps in Japan stories of Japanese barbarism surfaced. Though true, they were appalling beyond belief; we again counted ourselves, sincerely, among the lucky. Trials were held after the war to bring restitution for the vicious treatment of innocent prisoners of war, men and women alike. Yet for such perverse crimes against humanity there can be no vindication for the perpetrators; on their consciences their evil deeds will remain an indelible mark.

News of how close the war had come to Australia, via New Guinea, was unknown to us in Japan. The Japs had attempted to cross the Owen Stanley Range on the mainland after all. We were very proud to hear that our troops held off so many Japanese at Kokoda, so close to Port Moresby; a remarkable and heroic stand for which they are honoured in history. It seems the Japs were destroyed on all fronts in their efforts to occupy Australia, both openly and covertly.

When the Australians finally occupied Rabaul, on September the 9th, it was discovered that the only survivors remaining from the original captives of 1942 were the four men of the *Freezer* group. It was from information supplied by these four, Gordon Thomas, Editor of the Rabaul Times, and three engineers, Creswick of the Public Works Department, McKechnie of Pondo Plantation and Ellis of W R Carpenter's, that the Australian Authorities could confirm the names of the civilians sent away on the *Montevideo Maru*.

Towards the end of May 1942, there had been a muster of prisoners called by the Japs; since this was the first time the Rabaul citizens and, indeed, all male prisoners had been assembled together since capture, the *Freezer* group carefully recorded the names of their colleagues. When the official Japanese list finally surfaced after the war it was inadequate, due to the difference between languages and difficulty in translation; the recorded names provided an invaluable comparison in identifying civilians on board the *Montevideo Maru*.

The Japanese ruthlessly killed anyone giving himself up after the men were shipped away in June 1942. The Rabaul survivors told the Authorities of two known groups of civilians who mysteriously disappeared; and heading one of them was Mary's husband, Tom. A group led by Tom Goss and Vic Pratt, another well known planter, gave themselves up in the middle of July 1942. After being held in the camp for two weeks these six men were taken away in a lorry one day and never seen again. Towards the end of 1944, Bill Korn, of Pondo, and the team of dependable New Britain and New Ireland men, of twelve strong, also vanished without trace. It will be remembered that this group was retained from the beginning of captivity to run the power plant and do specialised jobs. The Japs discovered that they had been secretly recording the names of Australian and American airmen shot down and held in Rabaul prior to being shipped to prison camps in Japan.

No news of the fate of the men who were taken from Rabaul on the *Montevideo Maru* or our own ship was ever received in Australia during the course of the war. The Japanese had never responded when Australian Authorities sought information as to the whereabouts of prisoners of war from Rabaul. Not until the war ended and information was received from our group and the officers accompanying us on the *Naruto Maru* could a special investigation be carried out by Australia. The Japanese were forced to admit the inescapable truth; and the information about the deplorable loss of over a thousand lives was finally forwarded to Australia.

In November 1945, it was officially confirmed that the *Montevideo Maru* had been sunk by an American submarine off the Philippines on the 1st July 1942. The ship had no insignia identifying it as carrying prisoners of war. The official American Naval report stated that the *Montevideo Maru* sank in six minutes. Of eight hundred and fifty-three soldiers and two hundred and five civilians there were no survivors. Ironically, eighteen Japanese crew members reached safety in the Philippines. We travelled that same journey to Japan two weeks later and now, once again, counted our blessings on being sent to Japan and arriving safely, though only through sheer good luck, no one would deny!

The terrible disaster which befell those on the *Montevideo Maru* is little known, yet it was a monumental tragedy of the Second World War which has left lasting shadows of doubt in the hearts of many. The official announcement put at rest the anguish of over three and a half years of patient waiting, and a different sorrow, which would remain forever, burdened the hearts of hundreds - wives, parents, children and friends - whose loved ones were victims of the Japanese occupation of war-torn Rabaul.

Somehow I had known I would never see Noel again and had long ago resigned myself to the fact that there might be a day when I would come face to face with this reality. Pieces of the jig-saw puzzle, envisaged over and over, were quickly falling into place on my return home; but many pieces were lost forever and would never fill a place in the cryptic pattern of life. The joy of homecoming was touched with grief.

As the months passed many stories of escape from the Japanese invasion of New Britain in 1942 were, at last, able to be officially published. The rescue of hundreds of soldiers and civilians was successful mainly because of the magnitude of bush experience of Government officers, planters (including one lone woman, Mrs Baker of Langu Plantation in the Witu Islands), traders and missionaries involved; many active in the dual role as coastwatchers in those difficult days. After remarkable feats of survival in the jungle, avoiding Japanese patrols, parties reached Australia by sea months later - one small group as late as October. There were two large groups, whose escapes were carefully organised, and many small groups of individuals who took their chances on hazardous seas in not too seaworthy craft which, with a little assistance, doggedly steered a course to safety.

Demands have been made of the Australian Government over what was considered the abandonment of the Rabaul civilians; there were well over three hundred to give their lives over the debacle that beset Rabaul in January 1942. Mary's husband, his colleagues and lonely island coastwatchers were executed by the Japanese and lie in no known grave in New Britain with many more, slain while trying to escape. As mentioned in an earlier chapter the Tol massacre of soldiers and civilians is a principal example of Japanese brutality. And in the soul of a forgotten ship, in Valhalla, at the bottom of the sea, there rests a far greater number of New Guinea civilians with their brave companions, hundreds of loyal Australian soldiers of Lark Force and some thirty Norwegian sailors from the ill-fated *Herstein*.[1]

The trials of the Chinese population of Rabaul were simply expressed in a letter from Angela Choy who had been with us at Namanula: "Many hard times have I experienced since I see you before". The Chinese community had numbered about twelve hundred when invasion occurred and at the end of the war only eight

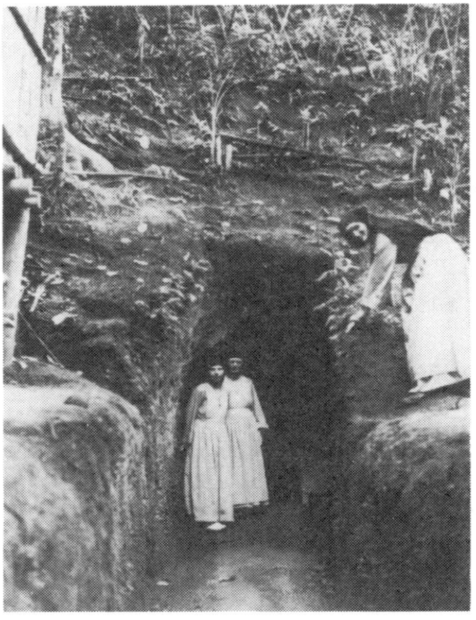

A tunnel at Ramale

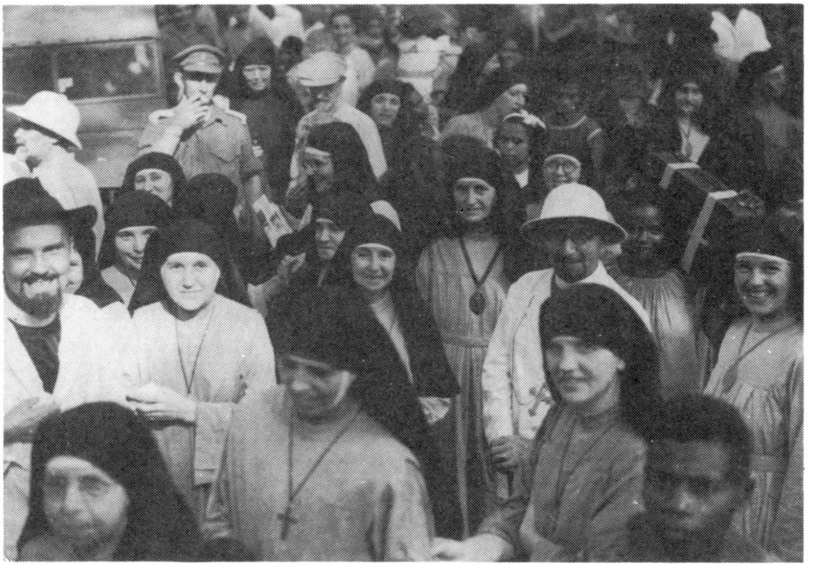

Missionaries with Bishop Scharmach (bottom right)

hundred and fifty remained. They were living twenty miles out of the town, and Angela told us that the Allied bombing caused all population groups in Rabaul to take to the surrounding hills and valleys before the town was totally destroyed. Angela did not mention the fearful cruelty of the Japs; the raping, looting and killing in Rabaul's Chinatown during the first few days of the occupation and no doubt afterwards, as the numbers remaining bear witness.

When the Japanese High Command made Vunapope Mission its head-quarters the missionaries were forced to live the last years of the war in Ramale Valley, inland from Kokopo. To be safe from the bombing they lived in tunnels dug into the nearby hills. The four civilians of the *Freezer* group were found by the occupation forces to be living at Ramale also. It was perhaps a miracle that they survived the war. Apart from our group and those who escaped, along with *recovered* prisoners in Japan (officers from the New Guinea Volunteer Rifles and Ist Independent Company of Kavieng and Doctor Watch), the *Freezer* group and the missionaries were the only citizens from the Rabaul area not to perish under the Japanese.

When the Mission was under threat of attack, the Japanese, too, were forced to live in tunnels dug into the mountains. The Allies found an unbelievable honeycomb of hundreds of miles of tunnels after taking back New Britain. Hundreds of Indian prisoners from the British troops in Singapore were brought to Rabaul to dig this intricate network. The Indians were treated appallingly by the Japanese as was evidenced by the condition of the survivors. Five hundred lie at the bottom of Simpson Harbour after the ship, whose hulk housed their number, was sunk during the blitz of Rabaul in March 1944. The Mission at Vunapope was razed to the ground by Allied bombing.

A letter from the nuns at Vunapope told of the death of Father Barrow. We were shocked to hear that he had died of amoebic dysentery, in Rabaul, towards the end of 1942, just four months after our departure. He had never complained of being ill, instead, his unfailing optimism and good manner cheered everyone; he had been such a wonderful help to us. There were many missionaries who died of disease during their internment or were killed from bombing in the later stages of the war. And yet more missionaries had been cruelly executed by the Japs, the Japs who said Christianity must be wiped out! However, ninety year old Sister Borgia was one of the survivors.

Joyce received by mail her gold watch, which she had left with one of the nuns when we were sent away to Japan. What a lovely surprise that it had survived the occupation, unharmed, hidden in a match box!

We hungrily read all articles in the papers about the war, of which there were many. Imagine our excitement on finding an article in the Telegraph about Geoffrey Lempriere (Ducky). It was written by the paper's special correspondent in Manila on the 14th September and could not reveal Ducky's name as his relatives had not yet been notified. He had only just been *recovered* from the now notorious Ofuna intimidation camp and was recuperating on a hospital ship in Tokyo Bay. The article told of his courageous exploits, while in prison, which saved many lives and many more men from torture. We witnessed first-hand his strength of character and were so glad to know he had survived.

A cheerful letter arrived from Cal who was in a South Australian hospital. The tuberculosis of her lungs was far advanced. She said she was feeling better and though nothing could be done to stop the progress of her illness she was glad she would die at home. Ducky had returned on the same hospital ship as Cal and she said that he was in fairly good health and would be getting in touch with us.

Joyce's Bill was the sole survivor of the boyfriends. He was discharged from the Army just after our return. Joyce and Bill were married in Brisbane a little later and I was proud to be Joyce's bridesmaid.

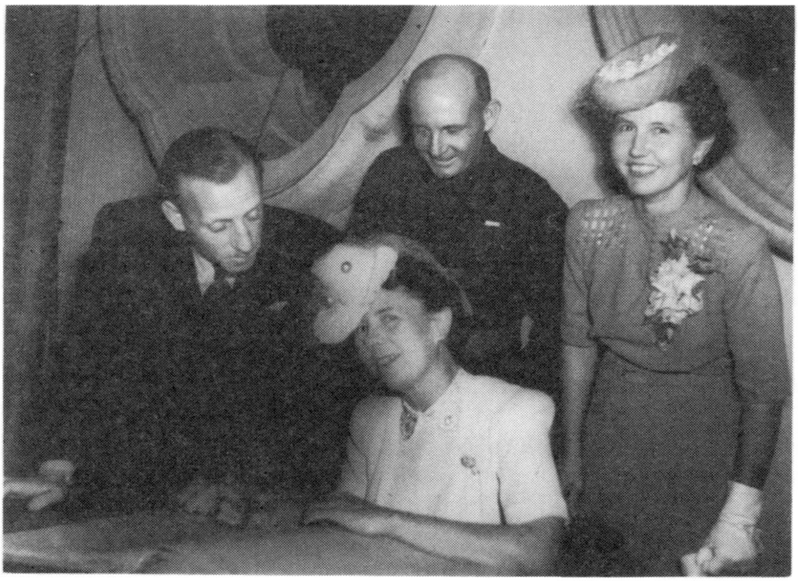

Happiness on Joyce's wedding-day

I remained in close contact with Joyce and Bill, and their happiness and the two children Joyce gave birth to over-shadowed bad memories of the War for the three of us.

A long time passed before we could feel normal people again. We found the most difficult part of fitting in was in communicating with people living an ordinary existence. There had been periods in Japan when some of us were scarcely on speaking terms with others in our group; yet now, we frequently sought one another's company. This insecurity slowly left us, as did the nightmares we all suffered. As months quickly turned into years in our up-to-date lives, a firm grasp was gained of our former selves.

When official letters arrived from Canberra offering renewal of our postings in New Guinea no one readily accepted. Time had not yet healed the wounds; and for most of us from the Administration Hospital there was no incentive to return to a place where happy memories no longer existed.

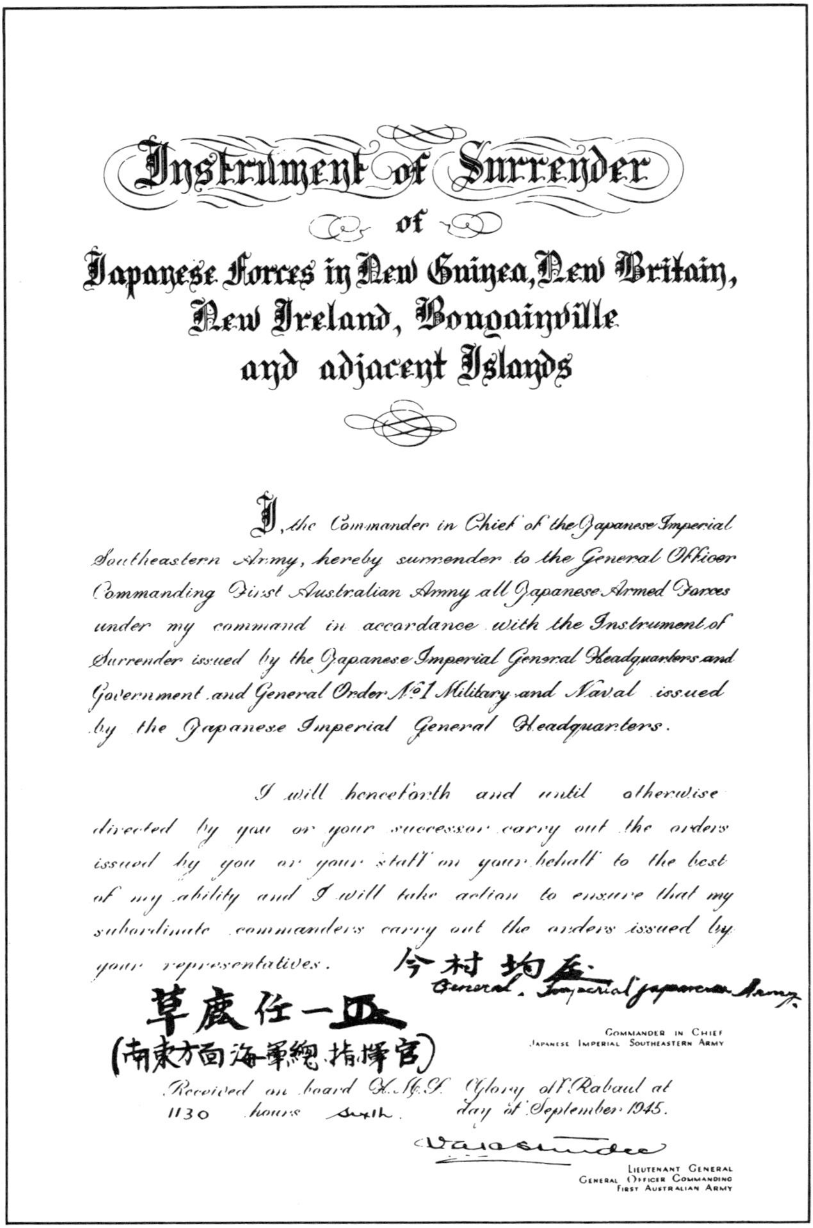

Instrument of Surrender

of

Japanese Forces in New Guinea, New Britain, New Ireland, Bougainville and adjacent Islands

I, the Commander in Chief of the Japanese Imperial Southeastern Army, hereby surrender to the General Officer Commanding First Australian Army all Japanese Armed Forces under my command in accordance with the Instrument of Surrender issued by the Japanese Imperial General Headquarters and Government and General Order No 1 Military and Naval issued by the Japanese Imperial General Headquarters.

I will henceforth and until otherwise directed by you or your successor carry out the orders issued by you or your staff on your behalf to the best of my ability and I will take action to ensure that my subordinate commanders carry out the orders issued by your representatives.

今村均
General. Imperial Japanese Army.

Commander in Chief
Japanese Imperial Southeastern Army

草鹿任一
(南東方面海軍總指揮官)

Received on board H.M.S. Glory off Rabaul at 1130 hours Sixth day of September 1945.

Lieutenant General
General Officer Commanding
First Australian Army

Surrender Document - Courtesy Australian Archives (National Office)

EPILOGUE

Fifty years have gone by since a beaten, devastated Japan surrendered to the Allies on 2nd September 1945. The world has forgiven the Land of the Rising Sun for the atrocious treatment of Allied prisoners of war, but no one has forgotten, least of all those who suffered. And indeed those who did not suffer must never forget the role Japan adopted in the Second World War, never forget the barbarism, for which there is no justification.

By the end of 1947 three Administration nurses and three Methodist Mission nurses had returned to New Guinea. Though not all stayed for a lengthy period they nevertheless made a valued contribution. Maisie and Oldroyd each gave twenty-five years of service, for which Maisie received an OBE; Dorothy Beale received an MBE for her twenty years of nursing with the Methodist Mission in New Guinea. New Britain saw the return of Mary Goss, a return to that place of very sad memories, especially for her; she died in 1953. Our friend Taffy Jones, though not a prisoner of war, made an outstanding contribution in New Guinea, eventually retiring in 1963, and Jean Christopher and Mavis Green returned to serve in the hospitals of the Methodist Mission.

New Guinea and Papua united after the war and became the Territory of Papua and New Guinea with the seat of Administration in Port Moresby, which fortunately was the only town not levelled by bombing. Full independence was achieved in 1975 and henceforth the Territory was simply known as Papua New Guinea.

In the Second World War Japan suffered its first defeat in history. In 1947 a new constitution was drawn up which, in theory, gave sovereign power to the people. The Emperor repudiated his divinity; and all form of Emperor worship was forbidden. A tradition which dated back to the transmitting of the three sacred treasures of the Sun Goddess to her heirs on Earth, the divine Emperors, was to be no more. The Emperor of Japan would never again be a living God on Earth through the Jewel of Nobility, the Sword of Strength and the Mirror of Wisdom.

Ironically, Japan was to gain from an American occupation following the end of the war. America took care, financially, of defence processes and enabled Japan to proceed unhindered with the prime task of building its economy. With technology adopted from Germany and America, Japan quickly rose from agricultural backwardness and a mediocre industrial output to technological and industrial prowess, mainly because of the dedication of the Japanese people to hard work. Devotion to hard work is considered a virtue among the nation's many cultural leanings. The Japanese have the most closely united society in the world, enjoying a culture which remains unique in spite of Western influence, and from which a mature nation with a sound economy has emerged. Today, Japan stands alone, no longer in need of alliance with America.

Where does Japan's future lie? We ask the question, and again much controversy surrounds the answer, which must surely unfold in the next decade.

In 1945 Japan was devastated by two atomic bombs and three and a half years of war and now, fifty years on, in 1995, the world sees a new Japan, a supreme creditor nation with economic and financial stability. Yet, after those fifty years, the world also sees in Japan a faction, which continues to linger, showing no remorse for the brutal actions executed during the Second World War.

As we advance towards a new Century, should we in the Asian region, and indeed the rest of the world, not hold some reserve in our judgement regarding the direction of Japan?

NOTES

RABAUL

1... There are six volcanoes which flank Blanche Bay and Simpson Harbour; three are extinct and three active. They are known by either their English or Tolai names. The extinct volcanoes are the tallest peaks of The Mother (Kabiu); South Daughter (Turangunan); North Daughter (Tovanumbatir).

The active volcanoes are Matupi (Tavurvur) and Vulcan (Rakaia). Rabalanakaia, with no English name, is a small dormant volcano beside The Mother.

The Father (Uluwan), lying on the coast south-west of Rabaul, is the tallest mountain on New Britain; it is also an active volcano.

2... The Frangipani Ball continues to be held on the last Saturday of May every year in the *new* New Guinea Club. The Club was gutted when Rabaul was destroyed by Allied bombing during the Japanese occupation, and, because of its unique architecture, it was rebuilt to the original plan and enjoys heritage status today.

During June, in Rabaul, the Frangipani Festival is also held to celebrate the town's revival.

In September 1994 Vulcan and Matupi (Tavurvur) again erupted causing widespread devastation to Rabaul and outer areas. The whole town was again evacuated to Vunapope Catholic Mission at Kokopo and the Methodist Mission at Malabunga as well.

In the interest of safety from predicted future eruptions, resources are being channelled to establish a new town at Kokopo - the origin of the first German settlement. Rabaul is being rebuilt on a smaller scale, geared mainly to foster tourism and port activities.

3... Kathleen I A Parker, Mavis C Cullen, Daisy C Keast, Eileen M

Callaghan, Marjorie J Anderson and Lorna M Whyte were the six Army Nurses detached to the 2/10th Field Ambulance Unit.

RABAUL - WAR

1... Flight Lieutenant B H Anderson, who was employed as a bank clerk in Sydney before the War, was killed in action on 22th March 1942, in a raid out of Port Moresby.

2... On 20th January 1942, seven Wirraways engaged the enemy. Two were already in the air on Patrol, which was maintained each day, and six took to the air when the enemy was sighted; one of these crashed on take-off. Twenty enemy aircraft were reported approaching from Tabar Island and thirty-three bombers came in from the west and were not sighted until they were over the town. Fifty more aircraft approached from the Duke of York Islands in the channel due east of Rabaul.

It was an impossible 'ask', but the Wirraway crews demonstrated unwavering courage in face of the enemy. Of the eight crews to contest the fight six airmen were killed and six wounded, two Wirraways landed safely with the four crew members unhurt.

3... Major Harold Page DSO, MC was a member of the well-known Page family from Grafton in Northern New South Wales; he had seen distinguished service in the First World War. Harold Page was married to Anne Brewster of Lismore and their gallant son, Robert Charles Page DSO, who died while a prisoner of war in Singapore only one month before the Japanese surrender, was a member of "Z" Special Unit. Harold Page was the Government Secretary and Deputy Administrator heading affairs at Rabaul in the absence of the Administrator.

It was at Grafton where my mother and step-father established a bus run after making their home at Brushgrove, nearby.

4... On receiving orders to attack the approaching convoy with his one remaining Hudson, Wing Commander Lerew caused some consternation among RAAF Headquarters staff in the Central War Room, Melbourne, with his now famous signal dispatched in Latin 'Nos morituri te salutamas' (We who are about to die, salute you). In Roman times, this was the cry of the gladiators before entering the arena.

Wing Commander Lerew and most of the remainder of his Squadron together with some civilians and Army personnel were rescued from Sum Sum Plantation on the southern coast of the island, by flying-boats from Port Moresby.

Later, after the fall of Rabaul, Lerew was shot down at Gasmata while on a raid over New Britain. He was reported missing, but was rescued by two local planters and arrived with them in Moresby nine days later and was soon in the air again. Wing Commander Lerew survived the war and attained the rank of Group Captain. He was among the first airmen in the Pacific to receive the Distinguished Flying Cross.

5... Lieutenant Commander Mitsuo Fuchida led the bombing raid over Rabaul on 22nd January and is reported to have said many years after the war ended: Rabaul had only a token garrison. He felt like a hunter sent to stalk a mouse with an elephant gun. Hoping to find an enemy worthy of the name, he discovered neither targets nor opposition. His bombers could not return to their carriers with a heavy bombload so he ordered them to jettison their missiles over the jungle. He felt deflated. A large investment in time, fuel and bombs had been wasted, none of which Japan could really spare.

Fuchida was also the lead bomber pilot in Japan's 'win beforehand' raid over Pearl Harbor and the bombing of Darwin raid on 19th February 1942.

This Japanese Commander became a Christian evangelist in America, devoting his life to Christ, in the years following the war.

VUNAPOPE - REFUGE

1... This baby survived the Japanese occupation of New Britain. She was the youngest of four children of Dr and Mrs Josef Schuy, who came to the Mission in 1935. Dr Schuy was the second Mission doctor to run the hospital at Vunapope and initiated many valuable training schemes. Sadly, a sister of this baby died of dysentery during the extremely difficult Japanese occupation years.

2... Doctor Watch survived the war and rendered invaluable service in the prison camps in Rabaul and at Vunapope.

3... In Japan, the act of urinating in public is called *Tachishoben*. There are of course, laws against the practice, but it is commonly encountered. Where it is done has something to do with the marked division the Japanese have between yours and mine - private politeness and public rudeness - and the fact that urinating is never done in the private garden but only in the public street. It is typically Japanese only in that it is performed more openly and more freely than in most other countries!

4... Major Palmer and Captain Robertson rendered invaluable assistance to the men, who took refuge in the bush and at inland Mission stations. Their efforts were highly praised by the missionaries, the soldiers and the sick of all races. At Vunapope, in the civilian camp, there were two Administration doctors, one Mission doctor and Doctor Watch available to attend the civilian and Army hospitals.

Major Palmer escaped from New Britain and reached Port Moresby in April, 1942. Captain Robertson was captured by the Japanese and placed in a prison camp. Orderlies, Corporal L A Hudson and Private R M Langdon volunteered to stay with the Army hospital at Vunapope. They were executed by the Japanese.

In 1950 five bodies were recovered from a burial ground found near Kokopo. They were identified as Army and RAAF personnel believed to be in hospital at the time of the invasion.

5... There were seven survivors of this horrendous massacre at Tol Tol Plantation on 4th February 1942, one died from vicious wounds some days later, the other six, who escaped separately, eventually caught up with their companions, recovered from their wounds and finally escaped from New Britain.

The survivors were: Pte W Cook, Dvr W D Collins, Cpl C Marshall, Gnr M Hazelgrove, Pte H J Webster and Pte A L Robinson, who was from the New Guinea Volunteer Rifles. Pte N W Walkley escaped initially with the aid of Pte Webster; he died on 1st March.

6... Not long after the Japanese occupied Rabaul, Bishop Scharmach, in an audience with the Japanese High Command, received a decree stating that only he would be allowed to deal with the Japanese in all matters, whether important or trivial. It is worth noting that after the Mandate was granted to Australia in 1921 all resident German missionaries were allowed to remain; the Australian government expected future recruitments to be non-German. The Most Reverend Leo Scharmach was to most people a German and had served in the German army in the First World War. The Japanese (with some limitations) regarded the Missionaries as allies.

The Sacred Heart Catholic Mission was originally founded in New Britain in 1881 by a French Order, the Most Sacred Heart of Jesus, and when the Germans annexed the area in 1884 the French lost jurisdiction over their Missions to Germany.

7... The Deification of the War Dead and the Japanese system of posthumous awards and promotions reveals an important aspect of the closely united society of Japan and the meaning of the Japanese claim to have an 'immortal army'. The spirits of all those who have laid down their lives for the Emperor are enshrined at the Yasukuni Shrine in Tokyo.

It has been said that in Japan one is born Shinto and dies Buddhist. The Shinto religion means 'the way of the Gods'; the worship of unseen gods and spirits of ancestors together with the powers of nature. With its enlightenment philosophy Buddhism is strongly linked with Shintoism; the two religions are not antagonistic, but live side by side in harmony. Buddhism, linked strongly with Confucianism, came from China via Korea and was introduced into Japan in the 6th century. This marked the beginning of a long line of cultural borrowings from China.

8... The Japanese had no respect for Christianity. The native Catechists who kept the people together were prohibited from holding religious service; prohibited from assisting the sick and dying people and giving religious succour at this time; they were not allowed to administer baptism, assist marriages or call the people together for prayers. In 1943 catechists were interned as this seemed the only way to prevent them from doing religious work, to which they remained faithful.

In 1944, as an example of Japanese authority, Peter ToRot, a Native Catechist from Rabaul, was executed by the Japanese for breaking the law banning religious activity.

In January 1994 in a ceremony in Port Moresby, the now capital of a united Papua and New Guinea, in the first step to Sainthood, Peter ToRot, the young catechist martyr born in 1916, was beatified by Pope John Paul the Second during his visit to the Pacific.

9... Captain J R Gray of Engineer Services was buried on the site of his execution. After the war, members of the War Crimes Commission visited the grave - the missionaries related the story and pointed out the burial place.

In Japan, Dr Chikami committed suicide - a doctor who could cut the heart from a living man but was too cowardly to face his own trial!

10.. At the peak of the Japanese occupation there were an estimated three thousand prostitutes in Rabaul. The Japanese brought them to Rabaul and quartered them in Chinatown. During 1943, with the continuing, worsening situation of the War, 'the Girls' were evacuated. Ironically, and tragically, the transport ship on which they were travelling was bombed near New Hanover in St George's Channel and not one of these 'comfort ladies' survived. Many years have passed since the War ended and it has recently come to light that many Korean women were pressed against their will into this service for the Japanese.

VUNAPOPE - CONVENT

1... The former editor of the Rabaul Times, Mr Gordon Thomas reported "Sister Borgia had more than once jeopardised her life to protect the younger nuns from the bombing from Allied air bases". Sister Borgia was among the Missionary sisters who survived captivity in New Britain.

2... Many visits were made to the islands of the South Pacific and the Australian Mandated Territory by the Japanese in the early 1930's and after the Second World War began. As early as 1934 the sailings of the *Heiye Maru* were reported as being a notable cause of concern, in 1939 the *Amano Maru*, while calling at various ports was described as 'a sinister looking craft'. The *Takaichiho Maru* ran four regular trips per year to Rabaul, Port Moresby and other island ports carrying insufficient cargo to warrant the expense, but placing her in an excellent position to keep an eye on Australian development in the Pacific.

3... There are over 700 native dialects in Papua and New Guinea, said to make up 45% of the world's languages.

4... The Japanese and the Americans both sustained heavy losses in the Battle of the Coral Sea. It could be claimed a *tactical* victory for Japan, but more importantly, it was a *strategic* victory for America. Japan was thwarted in her invasion attempt of Port Moresby and the severe damage caused to her carrier fleet handicapped Japan in the Battle of Midway, two weeks later. Midway was won by the Americans and this, Japan's first real defeat, was the turning point in the Pacific War.

5... The Naval Coastwatchers were established on the mainland of New Guinea, the Bismarck Archipelago and the Solomon Islands long before the Second World War began, with the aim to report unusual happenings, strange ships and so on. With the outbreak of war these stout-hearted men from all walks of life, Patrol Officers, plantation managers and owners - all experienced Territorians with a knowledge of survival in the jungle - volunteered to watch, report and avoid trouble. Their valuable information transmitted by teleradio, greatly strengthened the Allies and aided in winning the war; many of them gave their lives in this heroic work. On 8th March 1942, the Japanese brutally interrogated and murdered Percy

Good, a coastwatcher on Buka Island, after wrongfully suspecting him of relaying vital information. Immediately following this tragedy all coastwatchers were commissioned in the Navy, thus giving them combatant status.

Coastwatchers, supported by a number of RAN Signalmen, were operating on New Britain and New Ireland when the Japanese landed and not all escaped. Con Page, a plantation manager, is noted for giving warning to Rabaul of the Japanese raids. He refused to leave his post in the Tabar Island group when the Japanese invasion came, and four months later, after valiantly sending messages, he was captured with Jack Talmage, also a Coastwatcher. Both men were executed. Throughout the course of the war the coastwatchers could not have existed, wherever they were operating, without the loyalty of the local people. Page was betrayed eventually by natives who were swayed in their thinking by a German plantation manager on the same island. Ironically, the German, Herterich, was among those missing at the end of the war.

Assistant District Officer Keith McCarthy, coastwatcher, and an outstanding Patrol Officer since his arrival in the Territory in 1927, directed the successful evacuation of the 'North Coast' survivors, after the fall of Rabaul. Keith McCarthy was awarded an MBE at war's end.

Notable coastwatchers Commander Eric Feldt, the organiser, Lieutenant Commander W J "Jack" Read and many others were at one time New Guinea Administration District Officers.

6... The House of Mitsubishi is made up of two powerful financial and industrial families of Japan. It was part of a small group of influential families forming the Zaibatsu. The Zaibatsu had become so wealthy by the 1920's - largely due to assistance from Government policy - that it had great sway on Government. In 1924 the cabinet was called 'the Mitsubishi Cabinet' as it contained four members closely connected with the Iwasaki family of the House of Mitsubishi. The families of the Zaibatsu contained many ex-Samurai and shared the Government's expansionist policies.

After the Second World War the Zaibatsu combines were dissolved and broken up into component corporate companies. Westerners will recognise the Mitsubishi Zero and bombers among the many noted claims of achievement of this economically sound 'family'.

7... The strongest of the Buddhist sects in Japan is Jodo-shinshu, True Pure Land Buddhism, and is often viewed as a Japanese form of

Protestantism. The Amitabha, the Lord of Infinite Light, the Buddha in Mahayana Buddhism which began in the year 200 AD is the central being in the Jodo sects and is said to dwell in **Paradise** in the Pure Land in the West of Heaven. To those faithful followers Japan itself was considered Paradise, an extension on earth of the greater sphere above.

A SEA VOYAGE

1... The *Naruto Maru* was a 50 passenger cargo ship - she had no markings to signify she was carrying Prisoners of War.

The *Naruto Maru* met her fate on the 8th August 1943, when she was being used to ferry aircraft to Japanese land bases in the Marianas group of islands. Just north of the group, she was torpedoed and sunk by a US submarine .

Of interest, the two ships used in the evacuation of Rabaul also met their fate early in the war. When the Japanese bombed Darwin on 19th February 1942 the *Neptuna* was sunk, along with seven other ships; many lives were lost including the life of the Captain of the *Neptuna*. On the 17th June 1942, after one of the many bombing raids on Port Moresby the *Macdhui* was left a burnt out hulk.

2... The *Ramses* was a German ship which had been in Japanese waters since the outbreak of the War in 1939. She was used as a prison ship in Yokohama, holding persons captured by German raiders who were awaiting confinement in Germany; when Japan entered the war in 1942 all prisoners, whether neutral or otherwise, were confined in Japan.

THE BUND HOTEL

1... In January 1995 the most devastating earthquake in Japan, since 1923, struck the town of Kobe, south west of Tokyo. Thousands of people both rich and poor were left destitute and a figure in the multi-billions will be required to repair the mammoth damage to this highly populated, modern city.

2... The Franco-German Armistice was signed in 1940. The Vichy Government was set up in unoccupied France and continued, in theory, after the German occupation of the whole of France in November 1942. Petain, head of the Vichy Government, entered his government into collaboration with Germany. France had never really recovered from the depression and the national loyalty of extremist groups was always a serious question.

The Free French Resistance Movement was formed by those Frenchmen who accepted and were loyal to General de Gaulle as the leader of Free France. It is well documented that the Germans savagely repressed the French Resistance Movement.

In September 1940, a 'base rights' agreement in exchange for recognition of French sovereignty was concluded between Japan and French Indo-China when the Vichy Government appointed Admiral Decoux as Governor-General of Indo-China to replace General Catroux, who adhered to the de Gaulle regime. Japan used French Indo-China as a base for her drive through Malaya to Singapore in 1942. The French flag flying above the Consulate represented the Vichy Government of France.

3... At the turn of the century when Japan opened her country to foreign trade, laws were passed preventing the lower classes from appearing naked in the streets. The laws were to appease foreign modesty and were not always strictly enforced.

YOKOHAMA YACHT CLUB

1... The *White Australia* policy existed in name only surrounding the Immigration Act of 1901; it continues to leave its blotted legacy to this day. In the late 19th century the Labour party stressed a threat to Australian working standards which was clearly demonstrated on the goldfields in the 1850's, when so many Chinese flocked to the country to seek their fortune. They worked hard and skilfully, for so low a wage, it was feared they would displace Australian workman. In 1901 the new Federal Government of Australia passed the Immigration Restriction Act to limit excessive numbers of foreigners, mainly Asians, from entering Australia. The Act of 1901 was repealed in 1958 and a new act, The Migration Act of 1958, came into effect; it maintains that an immigrant entering Australia without an entry permit may be declared a prohibited immigrant and will be deported.

2... For the first time since 1916, the Melbourne Cup was held on a Saturday in 1942. The actual date was 21st November. Colonus won the race by 15 lengths on a very heavy track.

3... On the 30th November 1942, in Yokohama Harbour, the German tanker *Uckermark* caught fire and blew up; lying alongside her the German raider *Thor* caught fire and was destroyed. Also lying alongside was the SS *Nankin* - renamed the *Loitan* - she was sunk by this explosion as well. Ironically, the *Nankin* was *Thor's* first Indian Ocean victim, she was captured two days out of Fremantle *en route* to Colombo on 7th May 1942 and was taken in prize to Japan, where her survivors were interned as prisoners of war. There were four other victims of the German raider, *Thor*: two freighters sunk in the Indian Ocean and two tankers captured.

4... January the 1st, New Year's Day, is a national holiday in Japan and is regarded as a most important day. Happiness and prosperity are wished for the coming year and prayers are offered at shrines and temples. Homes are decorated at the entrance with plaited green rice straw, which is used in Shintoism to denote sacredness. On either side of the entrance hangs a combination of gate pine branches, bamboo stalks and plum tree twigs, which are symbolic of longevity, constancy and purity.

5... Messages were received by the relatives of a large number of civilians and military personnel held captive in Rabaul. Identification cards and letters were written by the captives and dropped from Japanese planes as bags of 'bombs' in the vicinity of Port Moresby at the end of April 1942. Though many were found, it is not known how many were lost. Those fortunate relatives who received a letter could only wait out the war with patience; the fact that no more letters were forthcoming as the war progressed did not cause any less alarm as the heartless reputation of the Japanese towards their prisoners of war had become well-known by then. The Australian authorities received no communication from the Japanese and it was assumed that the prisoners were being held on New Britain.

6... Flying Officer G R Lempriere was an RAAF Intelligence Officer and a learned scholar from South Australia. It was he who composed, in Latin, the now famous signal sent by Wing-Commander Lerew to RAAF Headquarters Melbourne.
(See RABAUL - WAR Note 2)

7... My jersey is still in my possession and amazingly it is as 'good' now as when it was manufactured!

8... The significance of the Cherry Blossom has become folklore in Japan. The blossoms have been deified by poets to capture the hearts and sensitivity of the Japanese people. They represent not only the manifestation of beauty in nature but in life itself. In full bloom the blossoms last only a short time. They fall on reaching the height of glory, demonstrating that what is beautiful in nature and life cannot last, but will be preserved forever in immortality. Perhaps Komatz, in a subtle way (which we did not understand and, in our position at the time, could hardly appreciate), was attempting to give us a lesson in Japanese culture.

TOTSUKA

1... A Buddhist memorial service for the repose of the soul of a deceased member of the family is often held in the home. Services are held every seventh day until the 49th day, when the soul is said to depart for the other world. On these days relatives and friends offer prayers while the Buddhist priest chants Sutras.

2... In Japan on Buddhist All Souls Day prayers and feasts are offered to the dead so that their spirits may be relieved from suffering. This ceremony is celebrated as the Bon Festival in mid-July.

3... The Battle of the Philippine Sea which began in June 1944 and ended with the capture of Guam in August was the greatest aircraft carrier battle of the War and destroyed Japan's dream of victory in the Far Eastern War.

4... In Japan, *Koromogai* is the name for the Changing of the Clothes ceremony, whereby on the 1st October warm clothes are officially worn and on 1st June a change to cool clothes is made.

TOTSUKA - WAR

1... At the end of October 1944 American forces began long and victorious campaigns to recapture the Philippine Islands. With the collapse of Manila on 24th February 1945 Japanese rule ceased. American landings continued on the numerous islands of the Philippines, still held by the Japanese, and by the end of April there remained only a few isolated groups of resistance on the main islands of Luzon and Mindanao.

The Americans landed on Okinawa on 1st April 1945 and bloody warfare prevailed until 3rd July when this Japanese island was in American hands. In this battle the Americans lost 36 ships and 368 were badly damaged.

2... These aircraft were the most advanced American carrier fighters of the Second World War. They were the Corsairs and were dubbed the Whistling Death. This fighter had a rate of climb of 4,000fpm and a top speed of 450mph. It first saw action in 1944 and by early 1945 the Chance Vought factory making them was turning out 300 planes a week.

3... After the war it was recorded that "On the 9th March 1945 United States bombers dropped 1,000 tons of incendiaries and razed over 15 square miles of Tokyo, killing nearly 84,000 people and rendering 1,000,000 homeless." The result of this raid showed that Japan could be literally bombed out of the war and invasion by ground troops might be avoided.

4... The Second World War saw the birth of the *Kamikaze* - Divine Wind Special Attack Force.

By October 1944 the Japanese Military leaders knew the war could not be won, but would not accept defeat. Admiral Onishi was put in command of the, all but destroyed, First Air Fleet over the Philippines and considered he had no option but to put into practice the appalling idea of a human powered weapon. Strong influence in the belief that their country was protected by the Gods gave the Japanese pilots faith in the outcome of this suicide mission and in their own immortality, likened in mysticism to the brief blossoming of the cherry tree. They tied around their heads the *hachimaki*, which was traditionally worn to give spiritual strength in the performing of an overwhelming task. Over five thousand *Kamikaze* pilots gave their lives in vain; although the American and indeed British losses were great, the 'Divine Wind' could not stop the Allies from Victory.

PEACE

1... The Typhoon season usually stretches from August to October but many severe typhoons have been encountered in July; no year escapes without several typhoons occurring. The American Fleet sustained heavy damage when it passed through the centre of a typhoon at the end of June and the intruder on the 22nd August, the tail end of the typhoon which came through Totsuka, delayed the US Fleet from entering Tokyo Bay.

MANILA

1... On 5th July 1945, General MacArthur announced that of four hundred and fifty thousand Japanese in the Philippines only thirty thousand remained.

HOME AT LAST

1... In November 1941, the *Herstein* participated in a search for Australia's missing naval cruiser, HMAS *Sydney*. The *Sydney* was subsequently recorded sunk off the coast of Western Australia; of her complement of six hundred and forty-five officers and ratings, there were no survivors. These naval men share an end shrouded in mystery similar to their army companions entombed in the hold of the *Montevideo Maru*. Ironically, the Norwegian sailors from the *Herstein* were among the one thousand and fifty-eight prisoners purportedly on board; in his book, *This Crowd Beats Us All*, Bishop Scharmach expresses doubt that the prisoners ever left Rabaul. The *Herstein's* Captain, Gotfred Gunderson, escaped when Rabaul fell.

BIBLIOGRAPHY

Books:

Aplin, Douglas, *Rabaul 1942*, 2/22nd Battalion AIF, Lark Force Assoc, Melbourne 1985

Bishop Leo Scharmach MSC, *This Crowd Beats Us All*, The Catholic Press, Sydney 1960

Buckley, K & Klugman, K, *The Australian Presence in the Pacific*, Allen & Unwin, Sydney 1983

Clarence, Margaret, *Yield Not To the Wind*, Management Development Pub., Sydney 1982

Cooke, John, *Working in Papua New Guinea 1931-1946*, Lara Publications, Brisbane 1983

Feldt, Eric, *The Coastwatchers*, Oxford University Press, Melbourne 1946

Johnson, R W, & Threlfall, N A, *Volcano Town*, Robert Brown & Associates, Bathurst NSW 1985

Kettle, Ellen, *That They Might Live*, F P Leonard Pub., Sydney 1979

Kojima, Setsuko & Crane, Gene A, *Dictionary of Japanese Culture*, Chopmen Publishers, Singapore 1989

Lambert, J L, *Handbook on Modern History*, F W Cheshire Pub., Melbourne 1966

Marcus, Alex, *DEMS. What's Dems?*, Booralong Pub., Brisbane, 1986

Moncrieff, A R Hope, Vol.1, *The World of Today*, The Gresham Pub. Co., London 1907

Nelson, Hank, *Taim Bilong Masta*, Australian Broadcasting Commission, Sydney 1982

Prange, Gordon W, *God's Samurai*, Brassy's (USA), Washington USA 1990

Rhoades, Weldon, *Flying MacArthur to Victory*, A & M University Press, Texas USA 1987

The Japan Culture Institute, *Discover Japan*, Kodansha International Pub., Tokyo 1987

Wood, F L W, *The Concise History of Australia*, Dymocks, Sydney 1944

Australia in the War of 1939-1945 Series: Australian War Memorial Pub.

Gill, G Hermon, *RAN 1939-1942*, Canberra 1957

Gill, G Hermon, *RAN 1942-1945*, Canberra 1968

Gillison, Douglas, *RAAF 1939-1942*, Canberra 1962

Gillison, Douglas, *RAAF 1942-1945*, Canberra

Wigmore, Lionel, *The Japanese Thrust*, Canberra 1957

BIBLIOGRAPHY continued

Newspapers, Magazines:
The Pacific Islands Monthly
The Rabaul Times
The Sydney Morning Herald
The Townsville Daily Bulletin
The Army News, Darwin
The Daily Examiner, Grafton

Archives:
Sacred Heart Mission, Kensington, Sydney
Australian Archives, Melbourne & Canberra
Australian War Memorial, Canberra: Orig. Documents & Transcripts
National Library, Canberra: Orig. Documents & Pacific Manuscripts